ETHICAL PRACTICE IN CLINICAL MEDICINE

The learning and practice of medical ethics in a clinical setting requires many of the same structures and dynamics as the learning and practice of clinical medicine.

In this study, basic yet controversial issues such as death and dying, truth-telling, confidentiality, and physician–patient relationships are treated in great depth – issues whose principles and complexities it is vital for the practising medical ethicist to grasp.

What renders *Ethical Practice in Clinical Medicine* original is that it first presents the theoretical sources of virtue ethics and then works through a number of medical ethics cases using the materials from the sources. In addition, it is the first book to address directly practical clinical problems from an historical perspective by using classic texts by philosophers such as Plato, Aristotle, Thomas Aquinas, William James, and John Dewey.

Because this text is designed to be used by the busy health practitioner, the theoretical material is kept clear, brief, and to the point. Similarly, application to the clinical cases is crisp and concise. Professor Ellos's new book will provide vital reading for all medical students and those studying ethics in philosophy.

ETHICAL PRACTICE IN CLINICAL MEDICINE

William J. Ellos

Case Studies by John Douard

London and New York

First published 1990
by Routledge
11 New Fetter Lane, London EC4P 4EE

Simultaneously published in the USA and Canada
by Routledge
a division of Routledge, Chapman and Hall, Inc.
29 West 35th Street, New York, NY 10001

Typeset in Linotron Bembo by
Hope Services (Abingdon) Ltd,
Printed in Great Britain by
T. J. Press (Padstow) Ltd,
Padstow, Cornwall

British Library Cataloguing in Publication Data
Ellos, William J.
Ethical practice in clinical medicine.
1. Medicine. Ethical aspects
I. Title II. Douard, John
174.2

Library of Congress Cataloging in Publication Data
Ellos, William J.
Ethical practice in clinical medicine/William J. Ellos;
cases by John Douard.
p. cm.
Includes bibliographical references
1. Medical ethics. 2. Medicine, Clinical – Moral and ethical aspects.
I. Douard, John. II. Title.
[DNLM: 1. Ethics, Medical. 2 Philosophy, Medical. W 50 E47e]
R724.E42 1990
174'.2—dc20
DNLM/DLC
for Library of Congress 90–8447

ISBN 0-415-05069-3
ISBN 0-415-05070-7 Pbk

For Myrna and Lynn

I am deeply indebted to John Douard, Ph.D., of the University of Texas Medical Branch's Institute for the Medical Humanities who provided the case studies for this book. His understanding of the issues and objective examples provided me with a constant freshness and excitement which I hope you will all share.

CONTENTS

INTRODUCTION: ETHICAL PRACTICE IN CLINICAL MEDICINE

The first two years of medical school are spent basically in the classroom in an academic study of the principles of medicine. Delineations are made of the structures of anatomy and organ systems. The facts of basic medical data are learned in great detail. Then comes a shock. The last two years of medical school, often called a clerkship or clerking, initiate a whole new type of learning experience. This way of learning and practicing medicine will continue on through the years of residency and specialization. It will be the basic method of on-going constant learning during the whole of the physician's life and practice.

To many medical students the reason for the shock at moving from classroom to hospital ward is that the structures and principles so precisely learned seldom so rigidly hold in actual cases. There are constantly anomalous elements which will not neatly fit into a schemata. Recalcitrant details plague precision. This is especially frustrating to the medical student who is almost by nature a perfectionist and often something of a work-oriented maximum achiever. As a pre-medical student such an individual made very few examination mistakes, agonized over those which were made, and spent long study hours making sure that such mistakes would not in the future occur. This same pattern held during the first two years of medical school. What a surprise to find that on clinical rounds lack of certainty and fumbling about are a constant daily experience. Yet the highly educated guesswork which informs the best diagnostic and prognostic procedures yields often seemingly miraculous results. Over a number of years, and eventually over a lifetime, the skills of clinical practice are acquired and an ease and efficiency in patient cure and care is developed. The actual practice of medicine is a highly skilled art of immense

1

complexity and often virtuosic intensity. It is learned through the trials and errors of daily practice in conjunction with a great deal of role modeling. One learns how to be a fine physician by watching and working with the best physicians. A sharing in the inner life of the master physician brings life and health to the patient.

The learning and practice of medical ethics in a clinical setting requires many of the same structures and dynamics as the learning and practice of clinical medicine. Practical ethical training must also, like clinical medicine, be preceded by extensive study of ethical principles, structures and systems.

This study of the theoretical aspects in medical ethics is highly developed with an abundance of primary and secondary texts. Basic issues such as genetic engineering, abortion, death and dying, truth-telling, confidentiality, allocation of funds are treated in great breadth and depth in the literature. Almost universally these topics are treated from the viewpoint of either utilitarian or deontological ethics. An essential grasp of the principles and complexities of these theories is mandatory for the practicing medical ethicist. But there are problems in the current study of ethical principles and their application to clinical ethics.

Utilitarian principles work quite well in application to large groups of people. The consideration of the greatest good for the greatest number illumines many issues of social ethics such as the allocation of funds, the regulation of research, the proper use of resources. These principles are not, however, so helpful in the individual situation when the patient is not being dealt with so much as a member of a larger society but rather as an individual very much waging a personal struggle for life and health. A great deal of theory changes face in confrontation with a suffering, worried person seeking help. The medical profession recognizes this personal dimension of the situation by insisting on the sacred physician–patient relationship. Even a spouse or child is with some reluctance admitted into this relationship and then only when circumstances force such an admittance. As much as possible treatment decisions are to be handled between the physician and the patient. The role of others is consultation and support.

In certain areas such as the breaching of a confidentiality utilitarian principles provide very mixed signals. Should a confidentiality be breached only in the event of the possible or probable harm to a number of individuals consequent upon the keeping of a confidence? Or might the harm to a single individual provide a reasonable ethical pretext? Since confidentiality is concerned not with the greatest good of the greatest number but with the individual good of the patient, it is not surprising that utilitarian guidelines are problematic. Truth-telling presents another problem for utilitarian ethics. A physician tells the truth to a patient not because there is a concern for the general good but because the specific individual good of the patient is at issue. This is not to say that general utilitarian principles are not of use. But these are of use as a more theoretical explanation as to why confidentiality or truth-telling are important. They do not provide answers to genuine clinical dilemmas in both areas. The challenges of ethical practice demand a more intuitive, skillful approach than the theory can provide.

There has been a tendency more to apply deontological rather than utilitarian theory to practical situations. A deontological, duty-based ethic would seem to deal more directly with the responsibilities of the physician in a concrete clinical encounter. Enormous use is made of W.D. Ross' principles of autonomy, beneficence and justice. The patient should be autonomous and the physician beneficent. The harmonious blending of the two duties might be justice. This distinction is greatly overworked. Moreover it is very simplistic. Ross himself provides the following highly complex presentation of what he called prime or *prima facie* duties.

(1) Some duties rest on previous acts of my own. These duties seem to include two kinds, (a) those resting on a promise or what may fairly be called an implicit promise, such as the implicit undertaking not to tell lies which seems to be implied in the act of entering into conversation (at any rate by civilized men), or of writing books that purport to be history and not fiction. These may be called the duties of fidelity. (b) Those resting on a previous wrongful act. These may be called the duties of reparation. (2) Some rest on previous acts of others, i.e., services done by them to me. These may loosely be described as the duties of gratitude. (3) Some rest on the fact or possibility of a distribution of pleasure or happiness (or of the means thereto) which is not in accordance with the merit of the persons concerned; in such cases there arises a duty to upset or prevent such a distribution. These are the duties of justice. (4) Some rest on the mere fact that there are other beings in the world whose condition we can make

3

better in respect of virtue, or of intelligence, or of pleasure. These are the duties of beneficence. (5) Some rest on the fact that we can improve our own condition in respect of virtue or of intelligence. These are the duties of self-improvement. (6) I think that we should distinguish from (4) the duties that may be summed up under the title of "not injuring others." No doubt to injure others is incidentally to fail to do them good; but it seems to me clear that non-maleficence is apprehended as a duty distinct from that of beneficence, and a duty of a more stringent character.[1]

Ross thus presents us with *prima facie* duties of fidelity, reparation, gratitude, justice, beneficence, self-improvement and non-maleficence. Yet the use of this tradition in medical ethics is almost always limited to duties of autonomy, beneficence and justice. A closer reading of the complexity of Ross' text reveals an attempt to deal much more in detail with the complexities of the situation.

It is precisely this complexity which has dictated a call for an ethic more attuned to the problematics of clinical practice. A somewhat impassioned plea for a new approach has appeared in two of the most critically important American medical journals, the *Archives of Internal Medicine* and the *Journal of the American Medical Association*.[2] The suggestion is regularly made for the adoption of a biopsychosocial model.[3]

Interestingly enough this model has in fact been the basic ethical approach in the long tradition of European and American philosophy. Plato stressed living in harmony with our psychological and social patterns and drives. Aristotle added a particularly biological dimension. The harmonious accommodation to the rhythms of these patterns is termed living a life of virtue. This because a virtue is taken to be a good habit and one must regularly as a matter of practically instinctive course be in harmony with biopsychosocial drives. While numerous figures develop various aspects of this virtue ethic in Western thought, one of the most sustained treatments is that of Thomas Aquinas.

Building on the Aristotelian legacy, Aquinas produced a highly nuanced study of the workings of prudential judgment in moral decision making. This practical working out of an ethical problem is augmented in the pragmatic writings of William James and John Dewey by specific methods for resolution of difficult cases and by a particular type of psychological theory which allows and in fact encourages a certain openendedness or incompleteness in moral decision making. For this second element they are indebted to the virtue-context writings of the Scottish philosophers who set out the ground in which pragmatism could flourish. Contemporary writers such as Gunther Stent, Leon Kass, Ernst Mayr and especially Edward O. Wilson explore the biological aspects of this pragmatic-virtue approach. The whole school of moral development anchored in the work of Jean Piaget and Lawrence Kohlberg provides rich material for the psychological dimension.

Alisdair MacIntyre's work on virtue centers on a cluster of writers such as Bernard Williams, Robert Nozick, Philippa Foot, James Wallace, Edward Pincoffs, Michael Slote and Edmund Pelligrino who are rapidly developing multiple social aspects of virtue ethics.

Because virtue ethics in a biopsychosocial approach is a radically pragmatic venture, it makes no real sense unless worked out in practical application to actual cases. The format, then, of this text will be to first present the theoretical sources of virtue ethics and then immediately work through a number of medical ethics cases using the materials from the sources. Because this text is designed to be used by the busy health practitioner, the theoretical material will be kept clear, brief and to the point. Too many massive texts in medical ethics remain unread and unused. Application to the clinical cases will be crisp and concise.

1

THE PLATONIC
FOUNDATION

While often presented as the ultimate philosophical idealist, Plato can better be understood as a rather thorough pragmatist. This is so for two reasons. The dialog form in which he always wrote was actually a way of dealing with a single or set of problematic questions by working through them. Seldom is a conclusion clear and lasting. Rather there is always the need to develop more clarity on the subject. Also, along with this pragmatic approach in each dialog, there is a more general pattern to all of the dialogs. The earlier dialogs are shorter and more incomplete, the later longer and more finished. The central dialog is really a collection of ten dialogs called *The Republic*. In these ten dialogs is the statement of the most absolute idealism in Plato. Our knowledge is to be somehow reaching the ultimate form or idea of truth itself. Our actions should strive to attain goodness itself. But while the earlier dialogs lead upward to this idealistic presentation, the later dialogs lead on downward to the complexities and details of everyday life. The whole sweep of the Platonic enterprise is not to reach some never changing set of answers to ethical questions, but rather to provide an idealistic frame in which to deal precisely with individual questions.

One of the most famous of the early Platonic dialogs is certainly the *Phaedo*. Here Socrates presents arguments why death is not to be feared. There is an early noting of the role of virtue. Ordinary people have the virtue of courage in the face of death because they are motivated by fear or dread. Also people who are temperate and restrained in their actions may be so because of a balancing of pleasures and pains. However, only the philosopher practices courage or temperance because of a knowledge of the workings of these virtues. Wisdom makes possible courage, self-control and integrity. This wisdom is a kind of moral purgation from lower and more base motives.[1] This is clearly a form of moral development ethics.

This need to be reflectively aware of the reasons for the development and practice of virtue is developed almost humorously in another early dialog, the *Laches*. Two distinguished generals, Laches and Nicias, remark on the bravery which they have seen Socrates practice in the field. All three are strong practitioners of courage, but none of them is able to define or explain courage at all. They make an interesting advance in methodology, however, in that they recognize that while it is impossible to understand courage as such, they might be able to understand specific instances of courage. Each time a specific instance of courage is studied, there is a realization that no specific instance will explain courage in general.[2] Tendencies to identify the part with the whole must be fought off. But while Socrates in this early dialog still holds out the possibility of somehow reaching an ideal knowledge of the virtue of courage in itself, the failure of the project is itself extremely instructive. A careful knowing of the parts and pieces of any project may be all that can be done. We certainly do not and probably will not know all the parts and pieces of the practice of medical ethics or of the practice of medicine. But the thorough knowledge of one aspect of medicine or of ethics may be quite enough. This would be especially true of the knowledge and practice of virtue. The development of any one virtue could mean in effect the development of all of them. It would just be a matter of a point of entry having to do with personal preference or talent.

While this might be true as regards the practice of virtue, Nicias is aware that it will not be true as regards the practice of medicine. The physician will know of the workings of health and disease, but not of the values underlying the enhancement of health or the preventing of disease. Questions are raised as to whether life or health are always to be preferred to sickness and death.[3] The practice of medicine, piecemeal as it is, cannot be a central unifying factor for the practice of virtue. The practice of a single virtue might, however, be a key to the practice of all the virtues, including the virtues of medical ethics. Perhaps this is why it requires so much time to extensively study medicine, but rather a little intensive time to study the virtue of medical ethics.

At this stage in his investigation of the virtues Plato is not yet ready, however, to settle on one single virtue as central. There is rather an early suggestion of what will become a classic formulation of the number of types of key central virtues. Socrates remarks that there are at least three parts to the practice of virtue: justice, temperance and courage.[4] If we were to take the whole exploration of the topic of virtue itself as in some sense a prudential action, then there is present here already the classic formulation of the four cardinal virtues of prudence, justice, fortitude and temperance.

A more important dialog, the *Protagoras*, underscores the importance of wisdom as the most important and central virtue.[5] While holiness is added to the list of virtues, the discussion is really concerned with the problem of there being a more central or unifying virtue. Protagoras claims courage as the central virtue.[6] But, since this is only learned by practice, it seems that it cannot be taught. Protagoras is, however, very much the champion of the teachability of virtue. Socrates has taken the other point of view. Now at the end of the dialog they seem to have reversed positions.[7] The question will dominate the next dialog. It also remains a most practical question for the teaching and development of medical ethics today. Presuming that medical ethics really can be taught, what possible methodology would be employed in the learning of this most practically elusive power?

Meno in the great dialog which bears his name asks Socrates whether virtue can be taught. In reply Socrates says that he does not even know what virtue is.[8] Responding to Socrates' plea for help, Meno provides a list of virtues. Socrates makes Meno aware that all of these virtues deal with temperance or justice.[9] He goes on to demonstrate that acting according to any part of virtue, such as justice, will be to act in general virtuously. Yet there still remains the question as to actually just what virtue itself is.[10] There follows one of the most famous sections of the *Meno*. Socrates questions a slave boy about his knowledge of geometry. This shows that all knowledge is recollection. This does not maintain that we recall something of a former life or state. It just means that we have knowledge as part of our basic make-up. The wise person will pursue ever more knowledge. Wisdom is the guide to right action. Wisdom may well then be the central virtue.[11] We must constantly wisely work at virtue. Virtue, then, is not an aspect of us which automatically works. Socrates explains this by saying that virtue is not a part of human nature.[12] He is also concerned to point out that virtue cannot be taught. The reason is that we cannot clearly identify the teachers of virtue.[13] But virtue might come to us as a sort of divine dispensation.[14] This is certainly rather vague. Failing to reach precise clarity on the question as to what virtue really is, the dialog ends inconclusively.

Consider the Socratic mode of posing these questions in relation to the practice of virtue in medical ethics. Might we take it that all people are by nature good? Does this not underpin the physician–patient relationship? There is the deep presumption that doctor and patient are working toward the same good goal of increased health. The wise patient and physician will work together for what is best. But indications are much to the contrary. It is difficult to know what is best. We tend not to see the whole picture. There may be reasonable care for one or another aspect of the patient's physical situation. There is seldom good care for the larger holistic psychological situation. What is of benefit to one or another of the physiological or psychological aspects may actually be a detriment to other aspects. Administration of drugs or therapies is often (and often rightly) resisted by patients. This resistance may be taken to be a bad thing in the patient. The patient may see the physician's action as bad. The basic presupposition of a nature somehow tending towards the good meets severe strains and stress. The practice of virtuous medicine is more of a struggle than a simple cooperative venture. And this is so in the best of scenarios.

Aristotle will remain more optimistic about the place of nature in all of this. Difficulties notwithstanding there will be a certain place for the ordering of matters toward good outcomes. Should physicians share in this optimism? Do you know physicians who indeed do? Or should we follow the lead of many physicians known to us who take such a cautious view of the workings of nature and the confidence and trust to be built on those workings as to be not only pessimistic but regularly downright hostile.

Some diseases are hereditary, progressive and terminal. These can be very difficult for a physician who is trained to cure disease. But nature doesn't always work the way we would like it to, and there may be very little we can do except offer patients sensitive care and understanding. In the following situation, a physician forgets that we can't always control natural biological processes, and lets his insecurities interfere with his relationship to the patient.

Bob Jeffries has been hospitalized with Huntington's chorea for over a month. Symptoms of Huntington's begin with personality changes, moodiness, diminished memory and judgment, leading to involuntary and uncoordinated movements, dementia, and finally complete loss of control ending in death within 10–15 years. There is no cure.

Mr. Jeffries' attending physician, Dr. Walters, has always had trouble with patients whom he believes will inevitably die a painful death. He has had an excellent scientific training and has never come to grips with diseases like Huntington's because they leave him feeling powerless, despite his years of training and experience.

Now Bob Jeffries is demanding more of his time and energy than he believes he can give. Dr. Walters has ordered tests, a series of treatments with L-Dopa (which can have disturbing side effects), and muscle relaxants, but he has been erecting a barrier between himself and Mr. Jeffries. Dr. Walters has been spending less and less time with him, and has developed the habit of holding only short, terse conversations with him. This behavior has intensified Mr Jeffries' moodiness and incites his already unpredictable anger. He asks one of his nurses if Dr. Walters has given up on him. In the end, Mr. Jeffries starts to withdraw as well, and his condition appears to the nursing staff to be a good deal worse than they had expected of a man in the middle stage of Huntington's.

Dr. Walters' anxiety in the face of a progressive, currently incurable disease is understandable. But his unwillingness to attend to Mr. Jeffries' psychological and social needs may have contributed to the worsening of Mr. Jeffries' condition, although there was nothing technically wrong with the treatment.

If virtue is some sort of wisdom, how is it to be taught? How do we know who are the very good teachers? Do some physicians just naturally teach good medical ethics to their students? Do we not often take it for granted that this is going on? Do a number of us simply assume that by doing good medicine we are teaching good ethics? How do you do and teach the practical arts of medical ethics?

Thomas Aquinas will maintain that virtue is preeminently wisdom or prudence. He will also say that prudence is in some sense a gift of God. Does this over-intellectualize virtue? Pragmatists such as James and Dewey will try to forge a new kind of knowing with practicality as its cardinal feature. Is the pragmatically skilled individual the highest knower? Physicians are among the most intelligent members of our society. They could not have got into medical school if this were not the case. Are they also possessed of innate practical knowledge? Are they therefore the best teachers of medical ethics? Should they be the only teachers of medical ethics?

An important debate in many hospitals today is whether or not to inform terminal patients that Do Not Resuscitate orders have been written. It is very difficult to resolve the ethical issues raised by DNR orders, and even very experienced physicians can differ with one another. In the following case study, the moral position of the experienced physician may be no better than that of the resident. Is his attitude pedagogically appropriate?

Martha Williams, 77 years old, had suffered two cardiac arrests. Dr. Halker, her attending physician, believed she could not survive a third attack. He intended to write a Do Not Resuscitate (DNR) order for her, and was strongly opposed to discussing such an order with his patients. Since the hospital was currently in the middle of a controversial debate over their policy on getting informed consent for DNR orders, decisions were being made on a case by case basis. That Wednesday, during morning report, Dr. Halker and the resident assigned to Mrs. Williams' case had the following exchange:

R: Doesn't the patient have a right to know that she will not be revived if she has another arrest?

Dr. H: Mrs. Williams is very weak and very frightened at this point. We must empathize with her and try to understand how she would feel if we told her. Don't you think she would be even more frightened than she is already? And would that be a kind thing for us to do?

R: But I know how things work around here. A DNR would, in effect, be like declaring her dead. She would be put at a distance from the sources of care, so her care would diminish.

Dr. H: That would be wrong, of course, and we have to make sure she continues to get the best treatment possible. But don't you see that the damage we can do by telling her outweighs any moral rules about paternalism? And it's beyond anyone's control at this point. There would be no point in resuscitating Mrs. Williams, and that is all we could tell her.

R: You talk about empathy, but are you really trying to put yourself in her shoes? This isn't just a matter of "following moral rules" or respecting Mrs. Williams' rights in an abstract sense. We can try to feel her pain and fear, but we have to *see* her as a mature woman who may *want* to know about the DNR.

Empathy is important, but sometimes distance can help us see what our patients need.

Dr. H: What this patient needs is a kind of parental care.

R: Perhaps she needs to know.

Do you think Dr. Halker's practical knowledge and experience gives him a special grasp of what his patients ought to know? Or can a resident, nurse, or even a bioethicist takes a perspective not available to some physicians on a patient's right to know that a DNR order has been written?

The central Platonic dialog, the *Republic*, is a pivotal point for almost all of the basic philosophical questions discussed throughout the entire Platonic corpus. It also presents these matters in their most ideal and lofty guise. The tentative questions of virtue ethics raised in the earlier dialogs will here be brought to closure. While the dialog, which is really a set of ten shorter dialogs or books, is well known for its views on theory of knowledge and the nature of reality, its context is ethical. The first book takes up the question of the lot of the just and unjust person. Is the state of one any better than that of the other? The book ends by maintaining that everything we encounter has a certain function. This function is termed a power or a virtue. Different things have different functions or powers. The virtuous function most proper to the soul is justice.[15] The practice of justice brings happiness. This because the soul is acting according to its highest excellence. Aristotle will make much of this aspect of happiness. Good medical ethical practice, especially in the clinical setting, has much to do with a feeling of happiness in decisions reached and acted upon. What is often termed conscience might well be seen as a feeling of displeasure with something done or not done. Might there really be such an in-built ethical monitor or guide? Do we appeal more to this than to any set of objective norms? Or are there also norms to which our subjectivity conforms?

Any attempt to reach any ultimate ethical norms must be undertaken by an individual who has certain virtues or character traits. Most important among these are facility in learning, memory, sagacity, quickness of apprehension, a youthful spirit and a magnanimous attitude.[16] Just what we look for in the good physician. But these abilities must be combined with a disposition to live a quiet, orderly and stable life. This combination of subjective qualities will enable a person to pursue the highest ideals of ethics. In two of the most famous passages in all of philosophical literature at the end of the sixth and the beginning of the seventh book of the *Republic* Plato presents this pursuit of ethical ideals as a pursuit of the ideal of goodness itself. Yet really this is idealism. Plato knows that we cannot ever completely attain to this kind of knowledge. He will give us in the dialogs which follow a much more pragmatic and practical approach to ethics. But the ideal remains. It is that pursuit of perfection to which physicians are so firmly wedded. It is doomed to perpetual frustration. All patients will eventually become injured or ill and die. Physicians die. But nobody much acts on that fact in the practice of medicine. They are rather Platonists. Health is the ideal. The good doctor always seeks it. It makes the practice of medicine true and good.

In a series of dialogs which follow the *Republic* Plato deals directly with the problem of the kind of reality which would accrue to such ultimate ideals as truth and goodness. It turns out that even considered in an absolute and ideal way they are found to not be final, whole or complete in themselves. Rather they are permeated by lacks and uncertainties.[17] Anyone involved in the pursuit of such ideals now would be engaged in a much more limited task, but such a person would also be much more realistic.

In the dialog which follows, called the *Statesman*, all this takes a specifically legal turn. Is it correct to obey an unjust law? If the law is not considered to be an ideal absolute then the problem is not so difficult. A specifically medical example is employed. Would it be wrong to force a patient to comply with a particular medical regimen? Plato does not think so.[18] It would not be a sin against true medicine or a breach of the laws of health. These laws are not absolute and strong enough to allow for such an offence. The practice of clinical medicine constantly involves the breaking of rules. Does the practice of clinical ethics involve an equal breaking of rules?

In the following case study, a physician who has lived his life by religious and moral tenets is faced with a situation in which those tenets come into conflict with his sense of responsibility to aid suffering patients.

Dr. Johnson is an internist at Memorial Hospital. He now faces a serious dilemma. He has always believed that under no circumstances does a person have a moral right to take his or her own life.

But one of his patients, Mrs. Harwood, is in the late stages of a very painful, terminal lung cancer, and he has been prescribing pain killing drugs, including morphine. She has developed a tolerance to all of them, and is in constant pain. She has asked him to prescribe a very large dose of one of the painkillers, and he has no doubt that she will use it to take her own life.

Complicating the situation, Mrs. Harwood has no family left. She is alone, and she has told Dr. Johnson that the pain she is enduring is especially horrifying since she knows she is going to die and there is no one to be with her in her suffering.

Dr. Johnson questions the legality of helping Mrs. Harwood end her life, even though she hasn't explicitly told him that is what she intends. But more importantly, all of the religious beliefs and the moral principles he has let guide his practice in the past stand opposed to euthanasia as a matter of *moral* law. Yet he believes he has an obligation to help end his patient's suffering, and Mrs. Harwood is certainly suffering greatly. To let her continue suffering strikes him as being in no one's interest.

What should Dr. Johnson do? How do we weigh rules against one another? Is the concept of a moral rule useful in a situation of this sort?

A solution of sorts is reached by re-assessing the role of the lawmaker. In the *Republic* such an individual tried to attain to the highest ideals. Here lawmaking is seen as sort of a weaving together of disparate factors. This is illustrated by a consideration of how different virtues interact. Moderation and courage must work together.[19] This is a harking back to the balance of the types of virtue which was seen in the *Republic*.

But an important development has occurred. The *Republic* presupposed that the interplay of virtues was in pursuit of an objective ideal of goodness. The *Statesman* has made this more objective ideal akin to or at one with the working of subjectively competitive virtues. The question of the objectivity of virtue has been transformed but not solved. It is a question which continues to haunt the practice of clinical medical ethics.

In the last years of his life Plato produced a really most astonishing text. The *Laws* is a set of ten dialogs or books. It is considerably longer than the *Republic*. It is meant as an ultimate change in perspective from the *Republic*. Yet it is one of the most unstudied and unread of Plato's works. Philosophers enjoy the pursuit of abstractions and ideals. They are *Republic* people. Physicians and lawyers are *Laws* people. The *Laws* deals in great detail with the precise and complex aspects of the workings of a state. There is no assumption that all will work out in an ideal plan. What works case by case is of more importance. Ultimate ideal wisdom and goodness is not rejected, but the concentration is on the practice of virtue in detail.

The harmonious workings of virtue will be developed by the acquiring of good habits. [20] The habitual nature of virtue will be one of the main themes throughout all treatments of this topic down many centuries. Aquinas is the thinker who will most identify virtue and habit. Others will seldom have the two long dissociated. Involved in all of this is a stress on the habitual virtuous building up of a good character. The good and virtuous person will strongly tend to perceive correctly what is right and to act on that perception. Problematic as this is for objective ethics, it seems pragmatically correct. Any practice skill demands a certain innate character or ability. We can and do build on this, but if it is not initially there, little can be done. One is born with artistic ability or not. There are born philosophers. There are born doctors. Are there born ethicists?

Ethics and morality appear to be in another category altogether. While we may be born with health, beauty or wealth, ethics is something we have more to constantly work at. Yet we are never happy unless we are virtuous. [21] Again there is the strong late Platonic stress on the interplay of the various types or aspects of virtue in the workings of a truly moral person. [22] Four virtues are to be especially interwoven: temperance, wisdom, courage and health. [23] This somewhat startling version of the four cardinal virtues gives a strong clue to the highly pragmatic character of this late Platonic thought. Prudence, fortitude and temperance are here. Justice is not. In its place is health. The earlier writings had placed justice as the central virtue. This led to the idealisms we have noted in the pursuit of ultimate justice. Plato seems to not be so interested in his later life in justice as in health.

A good deal of writing and discussion in medical ethics treats of matters of just distribution of health care resources. This is seldom an issue in clinical medical ethics. Health for the patient is paramount. Justice questions are subsidiary. Perhap Plato knew this long ago. The guardians or rulers in the state are not to be concerned with the promulgating of absolute ideal laws. Rather they are to be like military commanders, or like farmers, or like physicians. [24] All of these people deal with practical problems of the here and now. They must be able to diagnose the situation and do what is useful in a practical way at the right time. They fight not against injustice, but against disease, pestilence and iniquity.[25]

But Plato is ultimately very concerned indeed about the unity of purpose and action involved in the practice of virtue. Even though in this late period of his thought and work there is a concentration on multiplicity and detail, the earlier view of a transcendent unity of all things is not absent. How is the really virtuous person able to ethically educate if there is not knowledge of how the seemingly disparate elements of moral concern affect one another? The answer is at once pragmatic and filled with a sense of cosmic consequence. First we must be aware of the sovereign place of the soul in personal human experience. Given all that Plato has said about the soul, this means that one must have a radical sense of truthfulness to one's own inner ideals. The great Platonic example of this is, of course, the death of Socrates, who really brought about his own death rather than compromise his ideals. But now, even though Plato has been at great pains to show the problems of a too simplistic view of cosmic world unity, he again invokes the dream of a sort of universal mind among the heavenly bodies with which our own individual minds are in contact.[26] While this is a surprising and perhaps disconcerting move on the part of the aging Plato, it shows a number of the most pressing problems facing any theory of ethics. These same problems certainly face any version of virtue ethics.

At issue is the relationship of ourselves to any higher reality. Any inner personal set of virtues must somehow correspond to a larger reality. Our own personal lives and decisions must be part of a much larger scheme. At times all of us certainly have a sense of this. Always we find it extremely difficult to understand and articulate this sense. Physicians and nurses are aware on a daily and even hourly basis that their decisions have consequences of a life and death nature. What they say and do to their patients is regularly of the utmost importance in the way the patient views the situation of cosmic destiny. All matters of health concern make us aware of our limited time and resources. The experience of limitation itself seems to imply other aspects of reality not subject to the now perceived constraints. At least the limiting experience makes us aware of something or other, larger than ourselves, which produces the sense of limit or lack. We somehow run against some boundaries. In questions of life and death the boundaries can become clear and stark. Few would wish to embrace Plato's elderly advice to become in tune with some heavenly cosmic mind. But the question of ultimate validity and meaning remains. It is seldom absent from the hospital ward or the doctor's office. How do these questions impinge on the virtuous practice of medicine?

Bob was a well-liked patient, and during his 30-day stay in the hospital Ms. Williams, the night nurse, had spent many hours talking with him about the high and low points of his life. These discussions brought home to her the values that had sustained her through turning points in her own life.

Now Bob, who had AIDS, was dying of the strange diseases against which his immune system was helpless: Kaposi's Sarcoma, pneumocystis pneumonia carinii and neurological degeneration. There was very little she could do for him. But one night Bob held her hand and told her that he had just remembered something that had happened when he was a small boy, something that he'd forgotten. He had been daydreaming while crossing a busy street and almost been run over by a car. The experience frightened him and he sat on a stoop, shaking with fear. A woman who had seen the incident knelt down and talked to him. Then she held his hand and walked him home. That was all: but he remembered feeling like he'd just been returned to a familiar world after disappearing into a foreign land. And it was a stranger who'd brought him back.

The thing that struck Ms. Williams about the story was that it brought home to her just how strange she felt sometimes spending so much time with the very sick. But the connection she occasionally established with patients made her, too, feel like a stranger had returned her to a familiar human world.

Turning to the case of David, who became known as the "bubble-boy", the health care team and pastoral counselors who worked with him for many years had to reflect on their ethical responsibilities in the context of their sense of humankind's place in the universe. Given the technological accomplishment of the physician in charge of David's care, they did not all agree on how that technology should be deployed.

Dr. Raphael Wilson constructed a germ-free capsule or "bubble" in which David was placed when he was born. David suffered from severe combined immunological deficiency (SCID), which is an X-linked genetic disease transmitted from mother to son. Those who are born with SCID cannot resist infection, because the T-cells that provide cellular immunity and the bone marrow B-cells that provide humoral antibodies, cannot perform their immunologic function.

David's brother had died from SCID when he was several months old, but David lived in the germ-free capsule for 12½ years. This as an experimental procedure, and in effect David was a non-consenting human experimental subject. It was an extraordinary technological feat, but after 12 years David wanted out. He asked to have a very risky bone marrow transplant that, if successful, might allow him to live for a time outside the capsule.

He received a graft from his sister. It triggered uncontrolled B-cell growth in his intestines and he suffered fevers, bleeding, pulmonary and pericardial edema, and died of terminal arhythmia. He was 12½ years old.

Shortly before he died, David asked some of the people who had worked with him if his life had any meaning. The spokesman for David's medical team said: "David's life has been important for medicine but his greatest contribution was his death, because with this information we will be able to treat other children yet to be born."

This assessment of David's life seemed technocratic to the pastoral counselor involved in the case, and he argued strenuously that the medical team had performed an involuntary experiment on a human subject for essentially technological, rather than human, reasons. A moral principle that guides human experimentation is that informed consent be required from a patient before the experiment begins.

However, the ethicist involved in the case, who had known David during the entire ordeal and considered David his friend, expressed another point of view held by many on the medical team:

> "David's life expressed our hope, hope for a world that would one day be free from war, injury, and disease. That is why we gladly spent over $1 million on David's case . . . . David caused us to look at our own mortality and fragility. In a sense, we are all fragile bubbles floating on a precarious and tumultuous sea. The auto accident, the divorce, the loss of a job, the lump in the belly or breast can shatter us in a moment."

David's story elicited in all of the health care professionals who worked with and came to know him some sense of their place and limits in the world. Is medical technology a legitimate or an illegitimate extension of human limits? Is the sense of fragility and fallibility an important part of medical practice that can be revealed even in the context of modern medicine, or are we usurping the role of some higher power?

2

THE ARISTOTELIAN FRAME

The Greek mind was never far away from questions of ultimate cosmic significance. But it had also an extremely practical bent which wanted to contribute to the solution of the constant daily questions of life. Plato tended to place these questions in a larger context. Yet there is the noted trend in his later years to be more specific and particular. One of Plato's closest research associates of these later years was Aristotle. When time came for him to open his own research institute he tried to concentrate on the particular problems of living in the Greek world of the time. As will appear, the larger issues remain but the emphasis is quite different.

The Greek world of his time is the cradle of science, literature and politics as we know it. It is also more than any other time and place the source of our ethics. The various small Greek city-states with their often very divergent types of government provided a sort of working laboratory for ethics and politics. Aristotle knew this well. He really did have a flourishing research institute with a sizable team of expert scholars who set out to deal with the practical problems of the time. Their method was often to collect data from the various abundant sources at their disposal and then to let the data somewhat organize itself. Out of the very accumulation of detail a larger pattern or scheme might appear. One of those apparent schemes was the pattern of an ethic of virtue.

In the *Politics* Aristotle summarizes in a synthetic way some of the findings of his research institute. There is a very interesting section on the good management of one's household. Aristotle notes that it is much better to be concerned with the management of other people in the household than with the management of things. In both cases, however, it is important to concentrate on making sure that both people and things are maintained in as excellent a fashion as possible.[1] There is here already a strong clue as to the kind of more general order that interests Aristotle. The pursuit of excellence will be a key to clarifying the complexities we face. This is reflected in the very Greek word which we translate as virtue in the Aristotelian text. It really means excellence.

This pursuit of excellence implies and demands a hierarchy of things and values. While in this ordering people are to be preferred to things, some people are not much above things at all. One of the great anomalies of the free Greek city-states is that they had an extremely large slave population. But so did the American South before the civil war. What kind of excellence might a slave have? Should this term even be used of someone so low on the social scale? Would such a person be obliged to seek personal self-development for his or her own sake or only as an instrument of the master, part of a larger scheme of values and excellence? Can a slave have those excellent virtues of temperance, courage and justice? Aristotle's answer is clear and harsh. A slave has no deliberative faculty at all.[2] Hence the slave would not be able to partake of an essential part of the four cardinal virtues. According to Aristotle a woman has this deliberative faculty, but has not the personal power and control to use it effectively. A child's prudential deliberation is immature. Excellence or virtue will consist in all doing their best at the level at which they find themselves.

More than most professions medicine is highly hierarchized. While we do not have slaves the lowest level of hospital worker is regularly the descendant of slaves. The nursing staff is overwhelmingly female. Do the physicians on top consider themselves to be virtuous and excellent when they see themselves as functioning at the apex of this hierarchy? Is there a particular set of virtues proper to the different members of the hospital or medical team? Is an intern or resident considered to have strong powers of prudential deliberative judgment? How are these powers developed? What is the role of age and experience? When does age become a debility rather than a strength? What is the role of power in the establishment of virtue?

The important role power, age and experience play in medical decision making can be illustrated with the following case.

Martha Lofton, a 20-year-old mother of two, entered Memorial Hospital with symptoms of Multiple Sclerosis. MS is a chronic, progressive neurological disease with symptoms that include loss of coordination, blurred vision, speech difficulties and severe fatigue. The resident who was assigned to Mrs. Lofton diagnosed MS and the next day came prepared to discuss the case during morning report. Part of the dialog that morning, which included the intern working with the resident and a teaching attending, went like this:

R: I don't think we should spell out for Mrs. Lofton all the details of her disease.

T.A.: Should we tell her now that she has MS?

R: Well, why don't we just say she has "neuritis"?

I: That's lying! What if she asks you what neuritis is?

R: We can tell her it's an inflammation of the nervous system.

T.A.: Why should we hide the truth from her?

R: Because I don't think she's mature or emotionally stable enough to handle the truth. She's already worried about her children, and I don't think we should tell her she has an incurable disease from which she will die, although we're not sure when. It'll just aggravate her symptoms.

T.A.: Dr. R, it's very possible that you're correct, but I've had quite a few MS patients over the years, and your strategy might aggravate her condition even more by being too vague. I tried the same strategy with a number of my patients, and every one of them demanded second opinions. When they found out they had MS, they lost some of their trust in my judgment and it took time to get that trust back. Some of them demanded additional tests, which were costly and unnecessary. But the main point is if we tell her properly, we might be able to help her deal with the chronic nature of MS, and she might be more willing to trust our therapeutic recommendations.

Power is incorporated into the structure of medical education in several ways, most notably in grand rounds and morning reports. Can power be used, not to usurp the power or autonomy of others, but to help relative novices to develop certain medical virtues (such as honesty)? Does an attending's experience work as a source of moral education? Alternatively, might the resident or intern have more experience with a particular patient? Would an experienced nurse, who has a great deal of clinical contact with the patient, be a source of information that a rigid hierarchical structure might stifle?

For Aristotle there is a kind of ordering in all things. We can constantly note correspondences and connections among these orderings. For instance, just as there are different levels and grades of people, so there are different orders or patterns within a single individual. We have both rational and irrational tendencies. Reason must rule.[3] There is, then, a very strong rationalistic tendency in Aristotelian ethics which will have to be corrected at various points so that emotive and voluntary elements can also have free play. One way that Aristotle has of mitigating an over-rationalism in this context is to note that reason should be exercised by different people in different ways according to their state and functions. Courage and justice would be exercised in different ways by a man and a woman. There is a rooting of ethics somehow in the nature of the individual and of the situation.

A certain kind of energy or dynamism runs through Aristotelian nature. Virtue is practiced in exercising power over other individuals. But this power must be properly exercised. The guarantee of this is that our minds are guided by thoughts and contemplations which are independent and complete in themselves.[4] There is again the stress on the rational aspect of human nature. The more we study and understand ourselves the more we will go along with the perceived tendency to govern ourselves and others wisely and fairly. This is quite a radically different view of matters from a good deal of contemporary ethics. A considerable amount of time is spent in modern ethical thinking in trying to very objectively weigh and balance conflicting factors in a fair and honest manner. This is especially true in political situations pertaining to medical matters. Costs and benefits, rights and duties are subject to almost endless analysis. Results are seldom satisfactory. Aristotle counsels another route. The individual who has cultivated a right habit of clear thinking is more likely to make correct decisions. Complexities will remain in any case. Perhaps the very attempt to eliminate complexity in ethics is ill advised. The challenge of ethics is precisely this complexity.

The cultivation of a right habit of clear thinking requires leisure. Philosophy itself is termed a virtue.[5] He probably has in mind something like the virtue of prudence. Courage is the virtue most needed in business activities. Temperance and justice must be exercised, but in different ways, both in activity and leisure. This rather creative use of the cardinal virtues can give some quite practical pointers as to the kind of ethical activity we should prioritize in different situations. There are times when we have the leisure to carefully and prudentially consider the many details and possibilities of a situation. There are other times, especially in the clinical encounter, when swift action is called for. Here prudential leisure is ethically offensive. In either case we must temper our aggressive action or justly and fairly use our leisure time.

The principle of informed consent is an example of a principle many physicians believe to be prudent, just and honest all things considered. But not all clinical situations allow the physician time to discuss a procedure as completely as she would like. A particularly vexing situation is illustrated by the following case.

Memorial Hospital has had for many years a policy that requires informed consent for transfusion of blood products. Dr. Williams, the chief resident, has always in the past considered that policy appropriate and in the long term interests of her patients. Although she's had to deal with emergencies before, none of her patients had refused to sign the standard form which requests prior consent for emergency transfusions.

One day a 43-year-old male patient presented with severe chest pains. He signed the consent form, but indicated he wanted no blood products because of his religious beliefs. The attending physician, who had known the patient for several years, told Dr. Williams that Mr. Weber had only recently become a Jehovah's Witness.

Several hours after being admitted, Mr. Weber suffers a cardiopulmonary arrest, is given oxygen, and started on medications that stabilize cardiac output. He has also begun bleeding severely from an ulcer and requires transfusions. Mr. Weber is extremely disoriented and cannot engage in the sort of conversation Dr. Williams, the attending, and nursing staff would prefer about the wisdom of refusing transfusions. In fact, they are concerned that Mr. Weber might die from lack of blood if they don't move fast. The attending believes that Mr. Weber's religious beliefs are not so internalized that he would have refused transfusions if he had known he would need them to stay alive.

Should the staff decide to transfuse Mr. Weber even though he is very likely to go into another, and perhaps fatal, arrest anyway? What would the courts conclude, if Mr. Weber survives and chooses to sue for a violation of his religious freedoms? What virtues would be tested in a situation like this, and which virtues should take priority?

For Aristotle all the dynamisms of nature interrelate and interact. The public patterns of action and repose correspond and grow out of personal experiences of activity and rest. Our more physical self is more activity oriented; our mind more toward leisure. But Aristotle's rationalistic intellectual bias appears in that bodily activity is to be ruled by the mind.

Certainly one of the most important and influential ethics texts ever written is the Aristotelian *Nicomachean Ethics*. Here an attempt is made to give a clear and systematic presentation of an ethics of virtue. Toward the beginning of this text Aristotle gives a rather full account of the structure of human experience. This falls into three areas. We have a strictly irrational aspect. This is the bodily aspect of us which has only to do with nutrition, growth and bodily preservation. It is termed the nutritive faculty.[6] Since it is in no way under the control of reason, there are no habits of virtue which can be cultivated here.

For all the real strengths of the Aristotelian position, this treatment of the body presents two serious problems. First, there is here mentioned for the first time the term "faculty." There will now be a strong tendency both in Aristotle and in his follower Aquinas to lump together a number of quite complex and disaparate elements into a sort of thing which is termed a faculty. There will be a great risk of over-simplification. Second, there may very well be some sense in which we can speak of the development of some physical motor habits. While these habits might not be virtues in the ethical sense if they were considered as operating only on their own, the fact that we knowingly and consciously develop them makes them partake in some way in the world of virtue. Also we learn more and more all the time about the interplay of body and mind. Any contemporary use of Aristotle will have to incorporate in a more integral way the bodily elements.

We also experience what Aristotle terms appetitive tendencies. These are basically irrational drives toward some desired goods. But these drives can in some degree be controlled by reason, so there are habits and virtues in this area.[7] Specifically there are two kinds of appetitive habits. One is manifest in the giving of advice, the other in reproof and exhortation. Inchoately these may be the virtues of fortitude (here termed liberality) and temperance. This very sketchy preliminary treatment of the cardinal virtues also indicates that our rational powers also contain two elements. One part of our reason tends to follow or obey the other part. In terms of the virtues there is a distinction made between abstract and applied reasoning.[8] The later Aristotelian tradition will develop these into the cardinal virtues of prudence and justice. Aristotle in

25

further development of these virtues in the *Nicomachean Ethics* will not place justice in the area of reason but rather with the appetitive powers. This is a most costly move showing perhaps his still strong Platonic heritage. There is no clear place for a theory of willing or volition in Aristotle. The later tradition will make justice the virtue of the will. In Aristotle the presupposition is that if one knows something is right, one will do it. At least there will be two ways of knowing, abstract and applied. This will be of considerable use in the practice of clinical medical ethics.

The absence of a theory of will also precludes strong motivational factors from being effective agents in ethics. It probably also slowed down considerably the development of theories of un-conscious motivation. Whatver motivational theory there is is relegated to the area of sense knowledge and so is not considered to be of such importance as intellectual knowledge.

Justice remains a very thorny problem in any Aristotelian virtue ethic. The attempt is made to treat it as some kind of subjective trait of character. One would have a proper disposition to rightly distribute such things as money or honor or to rectify any injustices in such areas.[9] Objectively problematic and highly complex factors are ignored. In fact Aristotle identifies a sort of universal form of justice as simply the general practice of virtue itself. As a result an ethical approach such as utilitarianism is strongest on justice questions as it attempts an objective calculus and organization of complex and conflicting ethical claims. Because utilitarianism is the most common ethic practiced in the United States we have been much better at writing about justice questions such as distribution of funds, forms of insurance and regulation of the health professions. The knowledge and practice of clinical medical ethics remains a small and highly controversial field. Fortunately justice issues do not so much reach the bedside. Rather each case is decided as much as possible on its own merits in the here and now situation with little regard for the wider political and social issues which form a sort of an ethical penumbra. With the advent of diagnostic related groupings and profit-making hospital and health care cooperations this picture is rapidly changing.

Under the Medicare DRG prospective payment system, hospitals are given a flat payment for each primary diagnosis. They have to pay the difference if expenditures on a patient exceed the amount specified for that patient's diagnosis. Perhaps more importantly at this time, hospitals are allowed a fixed number of "Medicare days" for eligible patients, and when they run out of days they are sometimes compelled for financial reasons to send the patient to another hospital once he or she is stabilized.

With that background, consider the following situation. Dr. Walker is a highly respected heart specialist at Memorial Hospital. One of his patients, Mrs. Evers, was brought to Memorial one evening with a myocardial infarction. During the night she was stabilized, and the next morning Dr. Walker took over her case.

He wanted to keep Mrs. Evers in the ICU for at least several days longer. Although stable, she was weak and confused, and still clearly very ill. He checked with Memorial's Utilization Review Board, and they told him the hospital had run out of Medicare days, and that Medicare would probably not cover the costs. They recommended she be sent to another hospital. When Dr. Walker called a Medicare representative, she confirmed the URB's assessment and seconded the recommendation.

When the resident assigned to the case asked him what was going to happen, Dr. Walker said this:

> "In this case we'll be able to give the care warranted by the severity of Mrs. Ever's condition. We're her physicians, she expects that much, and we owe her that much. But I have clout in this hospital. If you or another less experienced physician had to make the decision, you would be under a great deal of pressure to send her to another hospital. In fact, it would be a test of your courage to resist that pressure."

We may need a new theory of ethical justice which combines the subjectivism of a virtue ethics with the objectivism of a utilitarianism. Certain aspects of pragmatism which will be explored later on in this text may contribute strongly to this new synthesis. But at the moment there is still a great deal more to be learned from the other aspects of the virtues which Aristotle develops.

Aristotelianism and utilitarianism do have one central element very much in common. They both stress the pursuit of happiness. The right to this, enshrined in the United States' Declaration of Independence, insures our access to both ethical traditions. Aristotle sees the enjoyment of happiness as the goal of all virtuous activity. Possession of higher and higher degrees of happiness will serve as a guarantee that we are acting virtuously.[10] Aristotle has often been criticised for propounding a too hedonistic view of ethics. This is not quite the case in that happiness is seen by him as an ultimate goal toward which the practice of virtuous ethics strives. Paradox-ically happiness is considered to be in a certain way outside or beyond human experience. This makes sense when you realize that Aristotle is always interested in having final goals or aims toward which seemingly disparate elements tend. The organization is provided by the goal or end. Happiness in itself is rather like the Platonic good in itself. While it is an odd way to treat the matter it does establish happiness as an objective reality and so Aristotle's ethics is not in any real way a self-centered hedonism. There is one other very practically useful aspect to Aristotle's use of pleasure. A virtuous ethical action will be a good action insofar as I get a certain pleasure in doing this action. This type of reasoning will receive a very full development in the intuitive type of ethics developed during the Enlightenment known as moral sense ethics. We will look at it in considerable detail. For now it is important to note how in actual everyday ethical decisions so much does turn on how we feel about that decision. If there is a certain pleasure and satisfaction in taking a certain action, we are inclined to do just that. Aristotle tells us that such an action is probably the ethically correct thing to do. This is not for the mere reason that we get pleasure from this action but because this pleasure is a sign that we are in harmony with the higher goals or ends of ethics. Everything in nature is tending towards some ultimate pleasure or goodness. Here is the Greek spirit of hedonistic optimism at its clearest, and at its finest.

But Aristotle's development of his theory of the intellectual and moral virtues situates them at one remove from the natural courses of nature. Certain natural processes, particularly in the material world cannot be reversed or changed. We might call these the natural laws of physics or biology. In the human situation, however, we recognize certain natural powers which we can develop. Among these are the virtues. They are neither innately part of us nor contrary to our nature.[11] Rather they must be cultivated in order to grow and develop. Now a telling distinction is made.

The two types of Aristotelian intellectual virtue will grow and develop through teaching and experience. The three moral virtues will grow and develop through the practice of habit. Moral virtues are not here distinguished from intellectual virtues implying that the former have nothing to do with ethics. Rather moral means pertaining to character development. It is very important to note that only the moral virtues are acquired by regular and constant repetition of the right kind of actions. The intellectual virtues are considered to be more abstractly mastered. These distinctions have direct application to a good deal of the experience of medical ethics, especially clinical medical ethics.

Pre-medical education and the first two years of medical school are concerned with what Aristotle would term the intellectual virtues. It is not repetitive habitual knowledge which is sought but exhaustive and precise knowledge of a vast range of biological, physiological and medical data. Seldom is the same material repeated in lecture or examination. There really is no time for repetition. The years of clerking and residency are just the opposite. Even though there is rotation among the various services, the same or similar cases are repeated over and over again. Skill is developed by achieving an ease and facility in dealing with analogous situations and cases.

Questions arise here not only about the teaching of medicine but also about the teaching and learning of medical ethics. Must there be a strong intellectual base before a student be allowed to deal with practical precise cases and real patients? Aristotle would think so. I think his reasoning here very sound. But is there also the need to have on hands experience of a large number of specific clinical cases? This too is needed.

Consider the following situation, in which a surgical resident in a well-balanced program has to provide appropriate information to a patient about treatment alternatives.

Memorial Hospital is one of the few teaching hospitals in the country with a program of clinical ethics for its first and second year residents. In addition to the clerkship Dr. Harvey has taken as an undergraduate medical student, and his clinical experiences as a surgical resident, he has been attending ethics rounds at Memorial for a year and a half.

Mr. Phillips checked into Memorial presenting with angina pectoris. His electrocardiogram indicated that he was suffering from single-vessel coronary artery disease. The surgical attending recommended coronary bypass surgery to Mr. Phillips, but didn't discuss with him the possibility of a more conservative medical approach.

Dr. Harvey had spent his first year of residence in internal medicine and had treated patients with coronary artery disease medically before. He learned that many internists believe the surgical procedure offers no significant increase in life expectancy, but also that angina complicates the picture. In fact the main claim for bypass surgery is that it can relieve angina refractory to medical treatment with trinitrin and B-blockade.

But Dr. Harvey remembered a case he'd had about 10 months previously which was very much like Mr. Phillips' case. That patient had chosen surgery against the advice of the internal medicine staff, and was one of the small percentage of bypass patients who contracted nosocomial infections, and he nearly died.

Dr. Harvey's experience on the internal medicine service and his conviction that patients should, whenever possible, be completely informed about the relative merits of alternative treatments, convinced him that he had to discuss the matter further with Mr. Phillips.

Problematic in all of this will be the relationship between the intellectual and the moral virtues. Are they so mutually exclusive? Can you learn one set without the others? Should some medical and ethical case work be integrated into the first two years of medical school? This I think should be done. There is also the question of the two types of intellectual knowledge which Aristotle proposes. The second or more practical knowledge is very akin to the type of information imparted even in the first two years of medical school. We are learning medicine not for the abstract study itself, but to make it work. Selection of just what to teach medical students from the vast body of medical knowledge is made basically in terms of what will best work now. Should, as a result, abstract treatises on medical ethics be somewhat suspect in that they are too removed from the actual case situation?

Many, perhaps all, of these questions can only be resolved by a practical consideration in detail of precise aspects of intellectual and moral virtues. Aristotle is often accused of having a too simplistically rigid ethics. He is portrayed as seeing human nature as a very fixed and unchanging reality. To understand ethics we have only to understand the structures of human nature. Actually as regards the moral virtues Aristotle is much more cautious. He goes so far as to say that we get moral virtues first by our exercise of them, not by any in-built endowment of nature.[12] It is vitally important that we perform the right kind of activity.

The first guide provided for us in the practice of the right kind of habits is that we ought to avoid defect and excess.[13] This is closely connected to another often misunderstood bit of Aristotelian ethics. By not going to extremes we follow a middle path or a mean.[14] This has been interpreted to say that the center of the road or middle path is always the best. At its worst this would simply be a counsel to non-activity. Even at its best it would not seem to be very good ethical advice. It would seem to prefer a kind of indecision or non-involvement as an ethical ideal. Seen in the context in which it is here presented quite another interpretation seems possible.

In the practice of the moral virtues there must be a constant testing of one virtue against the other. This is a rather tense interplay and interaction. Too much temperance or too much courage lead not only to unethical but to silly behavior. Needed is a not so much a balance between these virtues as a creative playing of one virtue off the others. Far from a static natural activity the practice of virtue is a hit and miss affair of struggle and strife. We can never take direct aim at the mean in itself, but rather we have to incline sometimes towards excess and sometimes toward deficiency.[15] As a result of this approach Aristotle in his survey of the moral virtues provides many examples of virtues in creative tension. This is often interpreted to be a search for the mean between two virtues. Really it is just to show how one virtue must constantly be influenced by another in the repetitive activity that constitutes the building up of good habits.

In the following situation a physician has to balance several virtues: the disposition to tell the patient the truth, her responsibility for personal care of a patient who might suffer from hearing the truth, and a sense of responsibility to and respect for the patient's family.

Judy Meyers, a 59-year-old widow and mother of three, checked into Memorial Hospital for tests. She had been suffering intermittent colon pain, and the staff wanted to rule out cancer of the colon. While the tests were being processed, Judy's children beg the physician not to tell her if the tests come back positive. They claim their mother is terrified of cancer and would have a very difficult time dealing with the information if the tests are positive.

The physician finally agrees to the family's request, but under protest; the tests show that Judy has stage C2 colorectal cancer, for which surgical resection can extend her life anywhere from ten months to five years. Since the operation must be performed soon, the physician is inclined to break his promise to Judy's children, and tell her immediately. On the other hand, that could cause her harm.

One possibility he considers is that a psychiatric consult can often help patients deal with their fears. He has done that before in situations where he was convinced a patient had fears he couldn't deal with alone. What should the physician do in this case? Is there a rule that he can apply to make such a decision easily?

In order to make these acts specifically moral three conditions must be present. There must be personal knowledge of the situation. The actions must be recognized as being specifically ethical and so be chosen for their own sake. These actions must proceed from a firm and unchangeable character.[16] This last element will be built up more and more as the first two elements are exercised. Aristotle here makes the very strong point that no amount of study of ethical theory will make a person ethical. The doing is all.[17] This is an extremely critical point in the teaching and learning of clinical medical ethics. Often programs of medical ethics are content with one or another lecture course. It really will not do. There must be the regular and constant involvement of students on rounds in the actual process of decision making. The more they can be made responsible for the decisions taken, the more an ethical character will develop. To a great extent this does happen in the residency years when more responsibility is assumed. But ethics programs in the residency training years are often very slim or non-existent.

The tenuous state of the virtues is again stressed when Aristotle maintains that the virtues are neither passions nor faculties. Passions are feelings accompanied by pleasure or pain. These are too in-built and natural for Aristotle to consider them to be virtues. Faculties are capacities to do one or another thing. But the mere presence of such a capacity does not mean that we actually do anything worthy of praise or blame. The fragile situation of the practice of virtuous activity is simply termed by Aristotle a state.[18] We will see Aquinas being much more precise about this placing of the virtues in the human make-up. Aquinas will also have a more precise way of talking about specific virtues, including a more integral way of dealing with justice.

But while Aristotle's sketchy theory of volition leaves the question of justice unresolved, the assimilation of volitional factors to knowledge elements produces a very strong presentation of practical ethical knowing. The contemplative intellect would be involved in knowing truth and falsity. The practical ethical intellect is always concerned with truth as it is enmeshed in the experiences of desire.[19] The speculative or more abstract type of reasoning is concerned to know the first principles of things. There is a certain unrelenting quality to this kind of thinking in that once any of these principles is discovered, there can be no change in this kind of knowledge. But practical knowledge (often termed *phronesis*) is precisely about matters where there are no fixed and unchanging principles. Rather it is about things to be done in a more rough and ready way. It involves deliberations about what can possibly be done, the science of the possible.[20] But the stress is on the various ultimate modes of human desiring and acting. For this reason practical knowing is distinguished from the practice of art which is only concerned with making something. *Phronesis* is more radical than that. It is the attempt to knowingly act in the best possible human way.[21] It is, then, a science of opinions and beliefs. We have to go along with our best possible beliefs for acting well in a given situation. This element of belief will be highly developed in the intuitive moral sense school of ethics. We will deal with it later in this text.

It should be immediately obvious how much *phronesis* is bound up with the ethical practice of medicine. Medicine is basically and primarily a decision oriented activity. There is constant deliberation with one's self and with one's colleagues as to just what to do in a given diagnosis or prognosis. Absolute certainties do not exist. There is a constant wrestling with desires of self, patient, family, colleagues. Opinions and beliefs are pursued, tenaciously held and discarded. Medicine cannot be learned from a text or studies in a laboratory. It is learned in the doing. The doing is always highly ethical in that all medical decisions involve regularly at the most serious level the course of human desires and aspirations.

Aristotle says that we can understand the workings of practical knowledge by considering and studying the character of people we credit with having it.[22] His most telling treatment of character is his beautiful analysis of friendship. There are three possible objects of love or friendship: the good, the pleasant, the useful.[23] If we are friendly with another person because we find that individual useful to us, this is a friendship of utility. It is a basically selfish friendship as we are looking to the benefit to ourselves. (This is also one of the strongest critiques of a utilitarian based ethic.) There is a certain crassness involved in such a relationship. We might rather be friendly with someone because we find them pleasant. This also remains a more selfish kind of friendship in that we are concerned primarily with our own pleasure and satisfaction.[24] Perfect friend-ship would be concerned primarily with the good of the other person. It would be a genuine altruism.[25]

Pre-medical students not infrequently tend to be loners. They are very highly intelligent. They are extremely competitive. They tend to be perfectionists and workaholics. There is often not the realization that, beginning especially with the clerking on service ward duties of the last two years of medical school, the practice of medicine is an often intensely group activity. The activity is certainly very useful. Most students find it to be extremely pleasant as they get their first taste of their medical goal of patient care. At its best it is always concerned with the good of the patient. It is also for the mutual good of each other. The better the medicine practiced by each member of the team the more they all learn and the more the patient is benefited. Constant slippage occurs among the three levels of colleagueship.

Both students and physician teachers have an enormous utilitarian stake in the professional relationship. They need each other to be able to carry out effectively their respective tasks. This is sometimes almost humorously evident in that the patient is almost overlooked in the process of recital collation of medical data. There are even times when under the pressure of the clinical situation the patient can become an object of humor. I have heard the recital in a medical work-up of so many complexities in a case that the team broke out into laughter: a most self-conscious laughter not only because of the complexity but because the complexity was so useful to the members of the group as examples of many things to be taught and learned. There is a constant need to check one's motives so as to find out whether the real motivation is the utility, pleasure or the good of the patient. This is also an excellent situation to show the objective efficacy of Aristotelian ethics. If the motive is true friendship for the good of the patient, the chances are very strong that proper action will be taken.

Friendship with the family presents yet other challenges and opportunities for a virtue ethic. We are often counselled to obtain the consent of the family for difficult procedures. This is especially the case in termination of life situations. While it is always good advice to get such consent, it is often the case that the family is divided. This may be because of the different medical expectations of various family members. It may have to do with uncertainty as to any procedure. Often family members are reluctant to make any decisions at all. Tragically in termination of life situations a long estranged family member may arrive on the scene. A sense of guilt heightened by the impending loss may drive such an individual to demand unreasonable and futile treatment. Questions of seniority among family members regularly occur. The tense situation encourages the development of latent sibling rivalries.

There is little that is pleasurable in such a time. Any selfish motivation on the part of family members is much more directed at the relieving of pain. But they may be more concerned about their own psychological pain than the physical and psychological pain of the patient. A good number of utilitarian considerations may be brought into play. There is often much discussion as to what is the most useful and expedient thing to do. But even with all of these problematic aspects of family behavior there regularly shines through a tender, touching and tragic concern for the patient. The family is not in the best position to cultivate this concern. The physician or nurse can be of great service. This is because the health care professional has both the closeness and distance from the patient to be able to provide an altruistic perspective. Not involved as such in family politics, the physician can help to focus attention on cure or care of the patient. In most caes the family is greatly appreciative of this friendly aid. The clinically cold and aloof physician saddens an already tense and tragic situation.

Often a medical team itself assumes a sort of transformed sibling rivalry posture. This is especially true in the medical school setting. There is the rigid hierarchy of attending physician, residents and students. Each are in a different type of competition with each other. At its best this competition serves the patient very well as the best kind of service is provided. The competitive situation also regularly provides a strong bonding of the team members. Each is doing the best possible to solve a common problem, often a life or death problem. The elements of utility in the situation are obvious. Somewhat paradoxically this is also a pleasurable situation. Physicians and students find immense satisfaction in doing what they do best. This pleasure is an integral part of the effective practice of medicine. We do our best in the types of activities which are self-satisfying.

It is somewhat easy to lose sight of the good of each other on the medical team. So much stress is put on the complexity of the case that individual team members can become just providers of information and services. Outrageous demands on time and productivity are common. The overworking of residents at long hours has become a matter of national concern and in many cases scandal. Physicians tend to consider themselves to be made of iron. Burnout and other related problems are rife. There is a need to be concerned not for the utility but for the genuine good of each other. There is more than enough of a base of mutual respect and esteem in the profession to build some of the best types of Aristotelian friendships.

3

THOMISTIC PRUDENCE

In the Middle Ages Thomas Aquinas much developed two aspects of Aristotle's theory of the virtues. There is much more of a stress on the habitual character of virtue. The notion of practical wisdom or *phronesis* is sharpened to precision in the technical study of prudence. In the course of this development we are provided with a quite practical guide to the acquisition and use of virtue which is surprisingly modern. There is in the *Summa Theologiae* an extended section on habits and virtues sometimes referred to as a treatise on this subject.

Before outrightly stating that a virtue is a habit, Aquinas discusses at length the workings of habits themselves. He begins by noting that a habit is a human quality disposing us to do good or ill.[1] The stress is on the tendency moving us rather strongly toward one or another course of action. Here as in so many ways in his treatment of these matters, Aquinas strikes some salient chords in terms of our understanding of the rhythms of ethics. There certainly are times when we feel more disposed toward acting at our best. At other times it is a struggle to get ourselves into a good mood. The demands of medical practice require that we are always as much as possible in the former disposition. A bad tempered or sour physician just will not be able to perform well. I suspect that a jackhammer operator might not have to display such dispositional discretion.

We also experience our habitual tendencies as somehow reaching out towards basically what is good rather than evil. An ill disposition does not make us feel better; a good disposition does. So we experience habitual activity as striving towards the perfecting of the human situation.[2] Encountering a sour physician or sour patient is an early signal of a possibly poor ethical outcome. In ethics as in medicine the striving for an optimal outcome is not a luxury to be used or discarded at will. Rather it is central to the proper and effective practice of both. The only way in which this perfection oriented activity can be properly developed is in the actual practice of virtue. Pragmatism is paramount.[3] The strenuous activity which is the pursuit of virtue is also the practice of virtue. It is important that goals are set very high. We feel a sort of inner necessity or drive towards doing our best. This must be a constant ideal propelling us through the complexities and drags of daily practice.[4]

Inner drives are by and large experienced quite inchoately. We might experience a tendency to be kind and considerate of others, but this is often perceived to be rather a small and delicate force. We often have to struggle to bring it to effective action. Yet the very existence of the experience is one of those preciously deep ethical signals which provide early guidance for our actions. It is symptomatic of proper ethical action.[5] But ethical action properly understood requires the use of reason to nurture and develop instinctive drives. There is a need to develop and study theories of ethics. A symbiotic relation grows between instinct and reason.[6] Because our instincts are random and unfocused, there is a need to engage in a number of virtuous actions in order to build up over a period of time a habitual practice.[7] It would also seem the case that one would have to explicitly concentrate on the ethical aspect of these activities. The more knowledge possessed of ethical theory, the more explicit these activites can be made.

This is not at all different from the experience of acquiring good habits in the practice of medicine. First the basic principles of medicine are learned. Then a knowledge is gained of a specialty. We are still not in the situation of actually practicing medicine. This happens only when we are consciously treating patients in a specialty such as cardiology or oncology. The skilled cardiologist is more and more precisely aware of practicing good cardiology. Actions of medical practice become more habitual. There is also a danger here in that one can concentrate too much on one or another speciality. An oncologist might become too fixed on attempts to cure a cancer and so overlook or not enough emphasize other medical aspects of the case.

The same problem occurs in ethics. Thorough knowledge of one ethical theory often leads to its overuse. We become blind to other possibilities. Yet the theory must be put into habitual practice if it is to be ethics at all.

Both in medical ethics courses and in medical training itself patients' rights are often emphasized. A patient-centered, rights-based ethical theory is certainly a very important framework for developing habitual respect for patients as persons, but consider the following case.

Mr. M. is a 38-year-old single male with a history of end-stage renal disease secondary to an extensive history of IV drug abuse. He has been receiving dialysis at the hospital for which you are the clinical ethics consultant, and you have talked with him often during the course of his treatment. He has been in a drug treatment program for the last two years, and has been free of drugs for about one year. He confides in you that he has been very worried about HIV infection and has undergone anonymous testing at the state's test site. The test was reported to him as positive. You know that he has been living with a woman for the past 6 months and in response to your questions he acknowledges that she does not know about his HIV status. He is unwilling to tell her of this because she has been important in helping him "pull his life together" and he is afraid she will leave him if told. He indicates they often, but not always use condoms for birth control.

You know Mr. M. has a right to confidentiality, and you have a corresponding obligation to protect that right. The woman Mr. M. has been living with is not a patient at your hospital. Do you have any obligation to her? Does she have a right to know Mr. M.'s HIV status, and does his physician have an obligation to tell her? Finally, are there grounds from the perspective of public health to override Mr. M.'s preferences in this matter?

It is possible that too great a focus on a patient-centered, rights-based ethic can prevent you from considering features of this situation that are morally important. But if you don't regularly take patients' rights into account, you may not develop the disposition to act whenever possible in their interests.

The acquisition of a habit is no guarantee that ethical activity will continue. Habits are fragile and can rather easily be lost. Because we often think of ethics in terms of ethical theory, we may consider ourselves to be acting according to excellent ethics when we have mastered the intricacies of the theory. This occurs much when medical ethicists first take up their job in hospital or medical school. Physicians expect a certain type of ethical expertise. This is often expected to be displayed by an ability to crisply and clearly cite ethical sources. Rigorous argumentation is to be brought to bear on cases. Yet when precisely this is done the result is regularly physician dismay. The explanations appear too abstract. They are too remote from the complexities of the case. Ethicists may appear too sure of their positions. Unintentional arrogance appears.

Part of the reason for this is that the intellectual, abstract aspects of ethics are the elements which are most unchangeable. Much time is spent in the production and critique of rather idealized theory. In philosophical circles the best theory often takes the prize. But in medicine theory is totally at the service of practice. Practice is habitual and subject to gains and losses, to dramatic changes over time.

Aquinas is aware that at the most abstract level the possibilities of human knowledge are fixed by the constraints and strengths of the human abilities to explain and understand. Here there is little or no change. But he is also aware that at the more general level of more experimental knowledge great variation exists. Habits of knowledge must be built up. Once this is done the knowledge must be habitually put to use or it will atrophy. We can often remember the principles but the details elude us. Yet medicine is nothing if not details. Ethics is nothing if not details. So there is a constant need even at the more abstract levels of ethics for constant learning, re-learning and re-examination.

Ethics and medicine are not matters of abstract knowledge. Clues, hunches and intuitions are crucial. The skilled ethical or medical diagnostician or prognostician knows and feels which are the best leads. Emotive clues are endemic. There is a sense of what is medically and ethically better and best. Choices must be subject to both intellectual and emotional tests. And all of this mix must be regularly tested out in practice. The fine honed edges of habit can be lost by ignorance, choice or misplaced emotion.[8] The best place for the clinical ethicist to be working is the best place for the physician to be working. Not in the library, office or laboratory but in encounter with patient perplexity. The challenges of this situation will ensure the growth of medical and ethical knowledge, emotion and choice.

But how do we know that our practice of medicine and ethics is correct practice? Clearly not any and every activity will lead automatically to better medicine and ethics. The Thomistic answer to this is to maintain that habitual action must be in consort and harmony with human nature. What distinguishes human nature from animal nature is our powers of reasoning.[9] Insofar as all of our habitual actions are under the control of reason they are better habitual actions. There are some curious consequences of this.

Our emotions and even our powers of free choice are considered to be not what is distinctively human about us. In these areas we act animalistically. Clearly this seems wrong in that our emotive choices are every bit as human as any other of our activities. What does seem right about this analysis is that our human employment of emotion and choice is experienced as occurring in a much more universally deliberative intellectual frame. Animals appear to act more instinctively. We reflect much more on the almost infinite possibilities of our actions. But it is important to note that our human choices and emotions feed into our intellectual situation in providing drive and motivation to ever greater knowledge. What is unique to the human experience is not the dominance of intellect but rather the level of the complexity of human operation. This is heightened when we are exercising our set of complex emotive and cognitive powers in close interaction with another person who is also exercising these same powers. The more we can mutually engage the complexities of both parties the better the ethics we will be able to practice. Also the better the medicine we will be able to practice.

The more we can involve larger groups in the medical and ethical scene, the better our ethics will be. Ideally and practically the more we can involve nursing staff and family, for instance, the better the ethical and medical outcome. Yet many physicians in fact tend to follow Aquinas' more rationalistic model. This model is very hierarchical in that it places reason at the summit and subsumes other human abilities under it. In actual medical practice there is a great deal of "doctor knows best" going on. Because the physicians have a much better education about medical maters it is assumed that they are to take charge. This much in the same way that reason rules the other human faculties. Not infrequently in medical practice it is not the physician's reason which is the ultimate arbitrator, rather the physician's emotion. Many physicians know that ethically a certain course of action should be followed but cannot bring themselves emotionally to do it. Emotion rules the situation but it is not the complex emotions of the possible participants, only the sovereign emotion of the attending physician.

Mary Beth is a 74-year-old resident of a retirement home, where she has been for the last three months. She had suffered a myocardial infarction and had been taken to Memorial Hospital until she was stabilized. It was her second heart attack, but she is doing well except for a slightly erratic heartbeat for which she is receiving one of the newer drugs for arrhythmia.

The staff at the retirement home enjoy her lively conversation, and have let her attending physician, Dr. Michaels, know that she is no trouble to care for. Dr. Michaels himself enjoys his once-weekly visits with Mary Beth. During one of those visits, she tells him she has been reading about legal aspects of Do Not Resuscitate orders, and assures Dr. Michaels that if she is ever in a situation in which she may need use of a life support system for an indefinite period of time, she would prefer to be allowed to die. She has lived a long and satisfying life, and would not consider death to be an unbearable tragedy.

Her daughter and son have also expressed a willingness to let their mother die under such circumstances, but insist that they be consulted before any final decision is made.

One day Dr. Michaels is called by the head nurse at the retirement home because Mary Beth has collapsed. Her heart sounds are very erratic, her respiration is extremely shallow, and her skin is cold and clammy and has lost all its color. She is having a severe reaction to the medication.

Since her fibrillation had not been noticed immediately, the code had been called with just barely enough time to resuscitate, and the chances are high that she would require life support. Dr. Michaels knows that this is the sort of situation that Mary Beth had anticipated when discussing DNR orders. He also has reason to believe her family would probably support a decision not to resuscitate. But since he is emotionally attached to Mary Beth, and, almost against his will, aware of the possibility that he might be sued if he allows her to die, he orders the head nurse to start resuscitation. When she asks whether a DNR order would not be appropriate, Dr. Michaels tells her angrily: "Don't argue with me. Start the resuscitation procedure immediately, and I'll be there in a few minutes."

Did Dr. Michaels let his emotions (fear and attachment) determine his decision? Did he ignore the emotions of the other participants in the drama?

Of some help in the resolution of problematic cases is a certain self-knowledge as regards what type of action usually engages an individual. A variety of factors push us to tend to act more regularly in one way or another. One physician is more cheerful, another more somber; one more academic, one more pragmatic. In many cases others observe this better than ourselves. A check now and then of what is the basic stance we bring to issues will aid greatly in our perception of what kind of ethics we habitually do.

Memorial Hospital has had a clinical ethics course as part of its medical education program for about one year. The teaching attending most supportive of integrating ethics into the curriculum, Dr. Jones, has established the practice of discussing the ethical dimensions of cases during morning report. Some of the residents have expressed impatience with spending what they consider to be too much time on ethics, which they believe is adequately covered in the ethics seminar they are required to attend.

About half-way through the year, however, something interesting happened. A first year resident, who had been criticized several times for consistently cutting short the relatives of his patients when they asked him questions, began his presentation of a case one morning by saying he had changed his mind about the value of critically discussing ethics during morning report. This is what he said:

> "I've been treating Mr. Robinson for a severe skull fracture and I had intended to release him without any further discussion. But last evening his parents talked to me about Mr. Robinson's life style, which is just the sort of conversation I try to avoid. This was a simple case, and four months ago I would have brushed them aside (politely, of course). But this time I listened. What they told me was that Mr. Robinson has been abusing alcohol for the last seven years, and he has never acknowledged the possibility that he may be an alcoholic. His skull fracture was the result of falling down the stairs during a binge. When I asked Mr. Robinson about this, he admitted his parents were correct, and that he now thought he should deal with the problem and asked for my help. If I had not changed my attitude I would not have known that this patient's problems were more complex than a simple skull fracture."

Do you think the ethical "peer review" played a role in the resident's change in practice style?

A unique feature of human habitual action is our ability to make these actions even better. We do not experience habitual actions as mere mechanical or rote procedures. Rather the better we get at something the more we are dissatisfied with ourselves. Not that this brings discouragement and pain. Rather we sense a creative set of possibilities for development. There is an element of perfectionism to all human habitual action. It is for this reason that such action is so specifically ethically virtuous.[10] It is much to the patients' benefit that physicians tend to be strongly perfectionistic. The very limitations of the science and art of medicine demand ever more work at perfecting the profession. This kind of activity is not peripheral to medical practice but central. There are few cases which are simply completely routine. The challenges of the situation make constant demands for better treatment. Slippage in such maters is medically and ethically reprehensible. Human habitual virtuous action is inherently ordered toward greater efficacy and accomplishment.

Peculiar to the human experience of perfectibility is that we cannot conceive of the final limitations of our possibilities. There is always more that we can learn; always more that we can do. We seem to have an in-built tendency toward development. We experience ourselves in a constant situation of creative unease. If this were not the case we might not be called upon so much to be virtuous as the practice of virtue itself seems to essentially be the striving for constant improvement. This applies specifically to ethical concerns. If we find that our ethical decisions are becoming pretty much routine, the chances are quite strong that they are not very good decisions. Just as we must be dissatisfied with many areas of our development, especially with our development as medical practitioners, so we must constantly be dissatisfied with our ethical progress. This runs directly counter to basically conservative ethical practice. Conservatives often maintain that they learned ethics once and for all. Some will say that they learned it at their mother's knee.

The dynamic and developmental nature of virtue can be seen in that it really only exists in its activity.[11] There is nothing settled about it. It is only acquired by conscious well-directed activity. It is lost by non-use. This fits in very well with the whole practice of clinical medicine in that the more use is made of virtuous action the more growth and development takes place. Aquinas makes this explicit by noting that a virtue is a habitual qualification of our activity. By this he means to say that it is not a deeply settled aspect of our make-up. Rather it is much more ephemeral and subject to change. In order to make sure that virtue constantly develops we have to always strive to make sure that we are looking towards good ethical action.[12]

While this at first might seem to be rather pedestrian advice, it does not turn out to be the case as there are many times in the wear and tear of clinical practice in which we can turn away from the burdens of ethical excellence. One of the easiest ways of making this move is to not see the range and complexity of the full situation confronting us. There are regularly a whole range of social and psychological issues which contribute both to the onset of disease or illness and the progress of recovery. One way of not pursuing ethical excellence is to concentrate so much on the physical pathology or injury that other factors are not considered. It is as though the physician's only job is to be a technician and fix a particular physical problem. Yet the basic reason why medicine has been held in such high esteem is that members of the profession were seen to be highly altruistic individuals who were concerned about the wider human frame of reference. They were anxious to know something of the personal problems and stresses which contribute to the disease or injury. They showed personal compassion during treatment. They were concerned to know further developments in the recovery process.

A great deal of current medical practice remains very faithful to these ideals. There is still very much the commitment to excellence which these ideals enshrine. The profession is still rightly held in high esteem. But the very complexity of modern medical practice does make the pursuit of these ideals more difficult. It is easier just to concentrate on the medical aspect alone. Ways must be found to make sure that the quality of excellence in medical practice can be constantly enhanced.

Aquinas has a notion of virtue as an ability to make the best possible decisions. There is a strong sense of idealism involved. But it is an idealism that is geared as practically as possible to operation in specific situations. So he presents a virtue as a kind of power on the very cutting edge of the best of ourselves in actual practice.[13] Since virtue is an operative habit, there is the need to be constantly putting it into practice. The practice of medicine affords abundant examples of this sort of activity. More than most professions it requires that one be always at one's best. This because of the very demands of patient care itself, but also because of the enormous and constant development of medical knowledge. It would be the rare (and probably not so ethically sound) physician who did not feel a regular sense of guilt as regards performance in both of these areas.

Dr. Johnson has been monitoring the interns' work in the neo-natology unit at Memorial Hospital since 10 a.m. As a neonatology fellow, she has teaching responsibilities, as well as having to act as consultant on new cases. Somehow she also has to find the time to keep abreast of the latest literature in her specialty. At 6 p.m., just as she was about to head over to the library, she received a call from maternity. The Welch baby had just been delivered, by Caesarian section because of fetal distress.

He was born blue and not breathing, and he was limp. It took 20 minutes to enable the baby to breathe on his own. It was one crisis after another and Dr. Johnson and the residents on the unit worked through the night. The seizures were caused by lack of oxygen to the brain, but lack of oxygen in a hypoxic baby also causes damage to the kidneys, heart and liver. The baby was stabilized after state of the art treatments to support blood pressure, prevent convulsions and keep heart and liver functioning were used.

Once the Welch baby, who was now named Steven, appeared to be temporarily stable (Dr. Johnson knew that Steven would soon start to experience another series of crises), Dr. Johnson went to the library to look up an article in the current issue of *New England Journal of Medicine* on hypoxia in neonates. That was part of her job, and she took it as seriously as she did her teaching and consulting responsibilities.

At 10 a.m. Steven went into another crisis. He had turned blue and had a pulse of 170. Dr. Johnson immediately diagnosed pneumothorax – a ruptured lung. Steven returned to normal after air had been removed from his compressed lung.

At 1 a.m. Dr. Johnson managed to slip away for a bite to eat and a couple of hours of sleep. She fell asleep, angry and frustrated. She knew that the most difficult chore lay ahead. Steven in the best of circumstances had a 20 per cent chance for a normal outcome, but at 12.30 p.m. the ultrasound technician had brought in a depressing report. Steven had massive intracranial hemorrhage, probably caused by the pneumothorax and increased venal pressure. His chance of even surviving for more than two or three days has been reduced considerably. There are emergency procedures that can be done, but they will require permission from Mr. and Mrs. Welch. In any event, Steven's chances are small and the Welches and

Dr. Johnson are going to have to make some very difficult decisions. For all of her skill, dedication and energy, circumstances such as these make her feel enormously guilty.

It may seem irrational for Dr. Johnson to feel guilty and angry. But doctors are human, and like the rest of us they sometimes believe that if they only knew a *little* bit more, or performed *one* more procedure they might have saved a patient's life. And when the patient is a newborn such thoughts are even more painful. Can you think of some strategies that can help physicians like Dr. Johnson cope with feelings of guilt, frustration and anger? Do you think that physicians who don't have such feelings are better or worse than physicians who do?

Added to these factors is the increasing role of ethics in decision making. Considerable expertise is required to even have some sense of the ethical options available much less put them into practice. What happens is that in most clinicians' minds there is a remote or more usually proximate awareness of the ethical dimension of key medical decisions, but considerable lack of ethical precision. In practice as a result doctors often have devised for themselves some rather simple and absolute ethical norms. Some, for instance, will never shut off a ventilator under any circumstances. Others will always employ aggressive antibiotic therapy. My own experience as a rounding clinical ethician is that there is a strong sense of relief in being able to talk through difficult ethical matters with a competent colleague.

Some physicians refuse to terminate life, on the ground that any form of euthanasia leads to a "slippery slope" at the end of which the "ethic of the caring physician" will be replaced by an "ethic of the killing physician." But will such an absolute rule, even if it could be followed, cover all morally relevant aspects of cases such as the following?

Barbara is a 12-year-old girl who had a spinal cord transection as the result of an automobile accident. She is mentally alert, but she is totally and permanently paralyzed from the neck down and needs a respirator to breathe. She has been on the respirator for several months, and she is still extremely depressed. She wants to be taken off the respirator and allowed to die.

A social worker, psychiatrist, resident, nurse, the physician who treated her at Memorial Hospital's trauma unit, the bioethics consultant and her attending physician all met recently to discuss Barbara's situation.

S.W.: Barbara wants us to remove her from the respirator as soon as possible. Her depression hasn't lifted at all and we have to decide what to do.

A.P.: Barbara's an intelligent girl. I've known her and her family for several years, and their emotional pain over her condition is extraordinary. There is no chance that she will get any better, and she will probably have to stay on a respirator indefinitely. From a psychiatric point of view, what do you think is her future emotionally?

P.: Depression, of course, can be treated, both chemically and dynamically. But even so, it's hard to say what will happen in her case. From her point of view, she has no future to speak of. Even if she recovers temporarily, it is very likely that she will need continual help in adapting to life as it will be from now on.

B.: All of this sounds extremely expensive. Can Barbara's parents pay for indefinite physical and psychological therapy that may or may not be at all effective? Can the state pay for such care? The respirator will be breathing for her indefinitely and at great cost. All of these factors have to be taken into account.

T.P.: I have dedicated my own life to saving lives. A long time ago, I adopted a simple rule: As a trauma physician, I must do everything I can to help sustain a patient's life, and I must do nothing to jeopardize that life. I know that Barbara's case is out of my control now, but if her parents act on her behalf to have her removed from the respirator, I will do everything in my power to see to it that they are prevented from doing so. Doctors can't start thinking they have the right to kill, even if the patient wants them to. And costs have nothing to do with what seems to me to be a very simple ethical and professional principle.

B.: Perhaps you're right in claiming that costs aren't the issue in this particular case (although when *are* they the issue, and for whom, doctor?). But Barbara is suffering. That we can all agree upon. She wants to have control at least over this phase of her life. If we don't respect her autonomy, I suggest that we might be heading for a different sort of slippery slope. Under what conditions will we respect the autonomy of any of our patients? Even if Barbara is too young to make this decision, why shouldn't her parents be allowed to make it?

S.W.: We have no reason, certainly, to doubt her parents' sincere and reasonable desire to put an end to Barbara's suffering, and we have no reason to believe that would be acting contrary to her own wishes. Doesn't she have some rights in this matter?

T.P.: Of course, but she doesn't have the "right" to commit suicide. And, as health care professionals, we have an obligation to keep her from doing so.

N.: But don't our obligations also include protecting our patients from suffering any more than they have to? Barbara has articulated her wish to die during many of our conversations. She's a wonderful, bright girl who knows that not only is she suffering, but also that her parents are suffering. But she feels responsible for it anyway.

P.: But since she is so bright, I think we may be able to help her work through that part of her problem. I'm inclined to think that since some of her emotional difficulty right now includes taking on the burden of others, we should wait for a while. We should also discuss this part of her depression with her parents.

T.P.: I think we should make a final decision now! And we should decide to keep her on the respirator for as long as she needs it.

This decision isn't going to be made quickly. Can you see how morally complex Barbara's situation is? Can a simple rule be justified if it covers over too much of the complexity? Are discussions of this sort helpful in revealing to the participants more of the morally relevant factors involved in such tragic dilemmas than they might have been aware of at first?

Aquinas has a structure for virtue ethics which attempts to deal with the dynamics of this situation. While he thinks that ethical right and wrong is rooted in voluntary decisions of the will, he realizes that only an informed and educated individual is in a position to make proper decisions. So our reasoning powers also have a set of virtues of their own. But the kind of reasoning which informs practical ethical decision making in problematic cases is quite different from abstract or theoretical reasoning. In medicine there is a considerable difference between knowledge of abstract medical theory and ability to put it into practice. But Aquinas maintains that there is always a relationship between intellect and will.

In this so highly scientific age we like to consider our research findings to be as close to certain as possible. Yet we do not attain absolute certainty. While this is true of even the most abstract of sciences, it is even more so of the scientific aspect of medicine.

Conditions of the present state of our knowledge and of the constraints surrounding the methods and procedures of medical research make certainty here a practical impossibility. Rather we work by as highly as possible an informed guesswork. A highly voluntary commitment and dedication drive us to explore ever new frontiers of knowledge. Sometimes this works well in that new and proper discoveries occur. Sometimes the opposite happens in that an over-zeal or fixed expectations for certain goals blind us to the real facts of the case. Commitment to excellence is the glory and shame of medical research.

Aquinas terms this kind of relationship between highly motivated expectations and the realities of precise and certainly accurate scientific research, faith. While this term tends to be used more now in a religious context, it applies well to the situation of medical research. More than in perhaps any other area of scientific endeavor there is need for faith and trust in the best available results. Shortly these research reults will be put to the acid test in actual use on patients who are often in dire and desperate need. Faith and trust in abstract science blend rather quickly into practical clinical situations where faith and trust between physician and patient are paramount.

The actual application of abstract intellectual principles to real cases is called in the Thomistic scheme the functioning of the practical intellect. The virtue most in use here is prudence.[14] Since this is the virtue which most precisely blends intellect and will in actual practice it might well be taken to be the central virtue. If this is the case, then it might serve as a key way of understanding the ethics of medical practice.

Medicine is a serving profession. While it shares this role with a number of other professions such as social work, education or even the law it has perhaps even strong affinities to the clerical calling. Both are motivated by a kind of deeply felt inner drive. Pre-medical students often feel a kind of irresistible inner urge to become physicians. Even the rigors of medical school fail to dampen that desire. Residency puts it fiercely to the test and at this point some people do drop out of the practice of medicine. Doctors often speak of themselves as following a calling much in the way that priests, ministers and rabbis follow a calling. The religious and medical professions deal daily with matters of life and death. The preservation of health itself involves often ways of motivating the patient that partake of the style of the religious exhortation.

The successful pursuit of the medical profession, like that of the religious, involves a good deal of role-modeling. Prized is the highly prudential person. While a good deal of practical information can be theoretically given, there is no substitute for years of hands on experience. There are very good reasons why we tend to trust the seasoned clergyman or clinician. Crucial to the practice and learning of prudential judgment is a sense of timing. Also needed is a strong sense of dedication. A lifetime dedication to the profession produces practical prudential results. Often the greater and longer the dedication the better the results. This is because the driving force of the will makes us always want to do better. The will to strive for perfection constantly pushes the intellect to greater achievement. In the dedicated doing is the wisdom and skill. But not all inner drives are to be listened to and followed. We often feel tendencies which should be resisted. Aquinas has a rather crude scheme of human passions which modern psychology rightly calls into question. But its very simplicity makes it useful for at least a first approach to the ethical questions surrounding passionate activity.

There are two basic passions called appetitive powers. The first is the irascible appetite. These are the kinds of feelings and passions which upset us. They must be held in check or carefully channelled. Pleasant feelings and passions are associated with the concupiscible appetite. These two must be controlled and made productive.

Aquinas does not think that force of will can creatively develop these powers. Rather they have to be brought under the control of reason.[15] This approach to the matter has earned the criticism of being a too rationalistic ethic. This would be so if the reason alluded to here were primarily speculative reason. But since this is all in the context of a discussion of virtue where the stress is on the intellect-will combination that is practical reason, the element of volition must also be strong.

Of considerable practical use here is advice to recognize clearly the role of various types of feeling states in the practice of virtue. It should be becoming more clear that really any practical art insofar as it is a practice has elements of virtue to it. That is why, for instance, we talk about good and bad art and hold the artist in some way even ethically responsible. It is why every profession needs an ethics. The growth of business and legal ethics shows the awareness of this connection.

But medicine, like religion, because of the seriousness of the ultimate questions with which it deals, is taken to even greater ethical task. And medicine, like religion, is an area of intense and fierce feeling and passion. A good deal of the irascible type of passion is stirred up by the collegial nature of medical practice. It is dubious that the driven young pre-medical student perceives the stress of very close group cooperation that the learning and practice of medicine involves. Right from the start you have to learn and love to work closely with the team. You don't even get your own cadaver to work on. You have to share even that. The clerking years demand the cooperation of the attending physician, the residents and the whole health care team. (Do not forget the nurses!) And so on through residence and on into practice.

Tempers regularly flare in these situations. One reason is that just about everyone on the team is either a workaholic or perfectionist or both. There is also the pressure of never having enough time to accomplish what needs to be done. Patients may be uncooperative. Remedies often do not quite work right. Hospital policies may force unpleasant decisions. The government and insurance companies get in the way.

Mrs. Louis was a 92-year-old widow living with her 96-year-old sister when the latter broke her hip and was placed in a nursing home. Mrs. Louis managed alone for a few months with the help of her daughter, who visited almost daily, brought groceries and did the heavier housework.

Mrs. Louis was a frail woman in good health. Her only medical problem was severe osteoporosis which had resulted in a painful compression fracture. She was not demented (although occasionally forgetful), was able to perform all ADLs (activities of daily living – bathing, dressing, eating) independently and was capable of travelling out of her apartment if assisted with transportation.

One weekend Mrs. Louis had a relatively minor stroke and had to be taken to the emergency room of Memorial Hospital at 2 a.m. The ER was crowded that morning, and the residents and nurses had been working very hard for ten hours. When Mrs. Louis was wheeled in, one resident muttered under his breath, "Another gomer [get out of my emergency room]." Ms. Haffner, the head nurse who was standing nearby, overheard him and told him to just keep his mouth shut and work.

Mrs. Louis was stabilized by the next afternoon, and the attending physician came in to examine her. He had already talked to Mrs. Louis' daughter, who told him that she would not be able to take care of her mother at home even though her prognosis looked good.

The daughter had her own family responsibilities and worked full time. Furthermore, Mrs. Louis had recently left the burner of the stove on, and the daughter was afraid that she would need even more care at home after the stroke. It had been a frustrating conversation, because the physician thought he had offered some good suggestions that would mitigate the daughter's worries. He knew that Medicare would at least provide some home care, but he wasn't too sure about non-skilled nursing home care which was more expensive.

Indeed, when he later called the Medicare representative, he found out that Mrs. Louis' nursing care would not be covered and would cost about $28,000 per year. After her own resources were depleted she would be eligible for Medicaid. Also, the social worker he talked to said that it may take some time to find a nursing home for Mrs. Louis with an available bed. In the meantime, the administration would be on his back to discharge her when her Medicare days were used up. He shouted at the social worker: "You'd better find her a facility soon, Mrs. Williams, or convince Mrs. Louis' daughter to take her back home. She can't stay here forever." He apologized to Mrs. Williams a couple of hours later, but he knew that there would be a strain in their relationship for a while as a result of his losing his temper.

They did find a nursing home for Mrs. Louis, but clearly high pressure situations such as this put considerable strain on a medical team that must act cooperatively if they are to give the best care they can. Can you think of ways to mitigate some of the tension that can build up in a hospital?

The very love of medicine itself can also lay a few snares. There is that inner drive to excel. There is a need to have a strong sense of one's own self-esteem and accomplishment. There is the real and genuine love for the patient and desire to help. Problematic also is the dedication to the profession itself. Many physicians just cannot tear themselves away from the practice of medicine. It becomes more and more their whole life. Personal and family problems peculiar to the profession develop. Frankly amorous attractions leading to scandalous episodes are not uncommon in medical practice.

Needed and prized are prudential role models who manifest in the care and precision of their work and dedication the balance needed to practice medicine at its best. The practice of medicine is a passionate affair needing constant control.

We tend to see this kind of control exercised in some way by our decisions, by our will power. Problematic, however, in Aquinas' view is the role of the will. He tends to make it a more reactionary sort of experience. When our intellect perceives something as good, the will pretty much falls in line to choose that good. But, probably taking a cue from the two great commandments of the Judeao-Christian tradition, he notes that there are two areas where our reasoning powers are not able to precisely and neatly present things so that the will rather automatically chooses. The intentions of God are not clear to us. Nor are the desires and needs of other people. If we are to love God with all our heart and our neighbor as ourself, we need to develop virtuous patterns of decision making which put a priority on our constant practice of correct choice rather than on all the reasons which we can put forward for those actions. This means that the very action of strong choice must have a certain habitual character to it. The sorts of virtues which are thus linked are the most altruistic ones. In order to bring about the best exercise of our will, we have to be involved in the highest exercise of will power, the habitual practice of love. Love of God and love of neighbor are seen as the main elements of this exercise of the will. [16]

Love of neighbor is the practice of justice. As a result of this point of view, justice is viewed in maximalistic terms. It is vital to always be going the extra mile, to strive for the most, not the least, that one can do for others. This runs rather contrary to many utilitarian or even deontological views of justice which much more stress a rather minimalistic type of ethics in the area of justice. The emphasis in these views is on protecting the rights of individuals. There is a rather adversary type relationship set up even among the most liberal of these views. Love is not often mentioned.

Because of the high level of intellectual achievement demanded of physicians, one would at first think that they might be among the most rational of people. But a number of factors point in just the opposite direction. In interviewing pre-med students who are trying to enter medical school, one is struck by the kind of inner drive which they show. They almost desperately want to be doctors. Not often are they able to clearly articulate the reasons for the driven following of the desire. Questioning often clarifies that in some inchoate way they really do want to help other people. There is sort of an in-built altruism which will not be denied.

Over many years doctors have to regularly return to this rooted drive deep within them. It is very difficult to do well in the practice of medicine unless there is a real love for the job. That love must be constantly directed towards the patients. They are the only real reason for the practice of medicine. But the press of demands for professional advancement can blur this picture and force a kind of selfishness. The inner purity of heart and will must be nurtured.

The affinity of medical and clerical practice has been noted. Both professions must be altruistic. Both deal in matters of life and death. Both are powered by a sort of inner drive. But just as members of the clergy regularly need to take time off to pray and purify their motives, so the same should in some way take place for doctors. Generally it does not. Time is too crowded. Demands are too great. Stopgap measures might well be in order. It might be useful, for example, to set aside some time for reading of literature. This may or may not have to do directly with medicine. But in many areas of medical humanities it is becoming more and more apparent that literature is one of the best ways of expanding the heart. Also literature exhibits a curious sort of rationality. At its best it may not appear very rational at all. It is not amenable to clear rational analysis. At its best it speaks directly to the heart.

This voluntaristic aspect of virtue ethics also plays a very large role in the kinds of actions characteristically taken in critical medical situations. Seldom is there a concentration on minimalistic rights of patient or physician. Rather the opposite. We tend to look for what is the most, not the least that can be done. We think that justice is only served when we have done all that we can. In this way the profession is rather removed from the more calculating ethic of a great deal of the rest of society.

In many areas of our lives we make decisions on the basis of a calculation of the risks, costs and benefits of an action to ourselves or to those closest to us. If an action will affect people who are not close to us personally, someone we think of as a stranger, we sometimes appeal to abstract moral rules (e.g. the decalogue). But a health care professional may find himself or herself in the following sort of situation, in which no simple calculations will yield an obviously correct decision:

James was wheeled into the trauma center at Memorial Hospital, suffering from a gunshot wound in the abdomen and a blow to the head. The ER staff had stopped his abdominal bleeding, he was transfused and hooked up to a respirator. For six weeks he lay in the trauma unit under heavy sedation to prevent him from fighting the machines that were keeping him alive. Since James was indigent, Medicaid paid for his care.

At this point, the trauma team met to discuss what sort of treatment, if any, James would receive. The difficulty was that it looked as if he would be dependent on the respirator, IV, and catheter indefinitely, but a neurological examination revealed that his brain was still functioning, and occasionally he appeared responsive.

Attending Physician: James doesn't have any family or friends, and he isn't capable of making his own decisions. Can we say definitely that he has a right to further remedial care or can we morally justify removing him from the machines. If we do that, he will almost certainly die.

Resident: What is our legal situation? Can we be accused of murder if we remove him from the machines?

A.P.: That doesn't address my question. What are our moral obligations at this point, even if the courts were to allow us to stop the respirator?

R.: Look. James doesn't have any thoughts or feelings about the matter one way or the other. We need his bed, if we are going to help patients who stand a better chance, not only of surviving, but of improving.

Nurse: Even if it's true that James is cognitively and affectively unresponsive, and I don't think we can say that for sure, but even if we can, doesn't he still have a right to care?

R.: Not if he's so far gone he isn't even a person. There are other sick people out there who have rights too, and we haven't any reason to think James will improve at all. Furthermore, the costs to society are tremendous.

N.: I've spent more time with James than any of you have. When the sedation starts wearing off I've seen him blink in response to a question or sound in the room. He's still alive, and we are professionally, if not humanly, obligated to provide as much care as we can, no matter what the courts say and no matter how much benefit we calculate others may receive from making his bed and our time available.

A.P.: "Thou shalt not kill"?

N.: No! If it were only a matter of following a rule, we would really be in a mess. In some sense we may be harming others by not taking James off the respirator. I've been taking a course in the Medical Humanities Program on literature and medicine, and one thing I never really thought about before is this: there are

56

some situations in which we must make a choice, but whichever choice we make will violate some moral rule or have bad consequences for someone. This is just such a situation. I know that whatever we do will be wrong. But I still imagine myself in James' place, hooked up to those machines and unable to communicate. That must be awful. I would wonder what the people on whom I depend will do next. If I were James, I would want everything done that can be done, until I no longer had the capacity to wonder.

If you were involved in this conversation, what would you recommend? Does the nurse have a point that the resident is overlooking? Does the profession of medicine involve a commitment to expand one's moral imagination beyond questions about rights and their corresponding obligations? Can health care professionals rely on legal decisions to get them off the hook morally?

Aquinas makes a distinction which is of some use in understanding the way we actually put virtue ethics into practice. He maintains that there are two ways of having a virtue. One just gives us a certain aptness for doing things. The other is virtue more specifically taken in that it stresses the ability to rightly put into use in a habitual way the knowledge we possess.[17] Intellectual habits can really only be of the first sort in that knowing something does not guarantee that we will do it. But medical knowledge is of a very particular type in that the only reason for knowing about it is so that something can be done. There are, however, according to Aquinas various ways of knowing. One he terms understanding which is a knowledge of principles. The second is called science or the deductive reasoning from principles to conclusions. The third is wisdom or a more general knowledge of how the various parts of knowledge fit together in terms of the highest kind of knowledge we can have of first and ultimate causes of things.[18]

Derived from Aristotle these descriptions are in one sense quite out of date. But they have a certain bearing on medical knowledge. The first two years in medical school are much spent on acquiring knowledge of principles in such areas as anatomy, physiology, organ systems. In the final two years of medical school attempts are made to apply these principles to practical cases. Over many long years of medical practice beginning with residency physicians try to gain the requisite wisdom needed to incorporate as much as possible the myriad complexities of medical knowledge into some sort of a coherent and workable synthesis. So while the divisions of knowledge along these lines are time worn, they still may serve some sort of practical use in coming to understand the actual ways in which medical knowledge and practice operate.

There is a need at times to emphasize one type of knowledge over another. Too much fascination with the principles of medicine might make one a rather poor practitioner. Too much time spent in the press of practice may erode knowledge of principles. It is always difficult especially in this age of specialized medicine to keep in mind the larger picture of the patient's overall medical situation.

One point made about the nature of an art or skill is very helpful in understanding medicine. The proof of the good use of art or skill is in the actual quality of the object produced. If a craftsman can produce a fine piece of furniture then he has the skill or the art of woodworking. If there is no fine product, then he does not. Because of the great prestige surrounding the practice of medicine today we tend to forget that medical schools are really highly expensive and exclusive trade schools. We do not yet have very good methods of testing just how well students do on patients as they are still so much under the supervision of their professors. Residents are more tested but still under such supervision that mistakes can rather easily be picked up and corrected by attending physicians. So the young physician often only gets a sense of real personal achievement and skill during the years of private practice. As they are able to more and more successfully care for and cure patients they acquire more proof of their expertise and confidence in their capabilities. But this can only be accomplished by a habitual and almost intuitive practice of the art and skill of medicine.

But the mere practice of an art or skill of any kind does not mean that we are involved in any clearly ethical activity. In order to do that we have to bring into play some sort of intentionality in the work in which we are engaged. It is a somewhat curious feature in the area of art and skill that we tend to use moral terms to describe the products of these activities. So there is good and bad art. And often the badness involved here is specifically moral. People get extremely upset, for instance, at certain aspects of modern art which are considered by them to be so bad as to have been produced in some sense by a bad person who intended wickedly to provide something distressing and distasteful which we have to view and live with. Poor productions of plumbers and carpenters are often ascribed to bad will on the part of the craftsmen themselves. Bad people produce bad things.

In order to continue in the practice of medicine, you have to love what you are doing and you have to love the people for whom you are working. The intention must color your efforts or the chances are rather high that the quality of your work will slip. If one is concerned primarily with making money or acquiring prestige the focus on the patient will blur. One cannot be content with just the skillful practice of medicine as a trade but must be aware of the really ultimate reason for the art, the care of patients. The public requires of its physicians a sense of dedication and commitment which must be regularly manifest in the physician-patient relationship. We must be rather testing our intentions to see that they are centered on the right goal. This kind of bending of intention Aquinas calls the virtue of prudence.[19] We must explicitly intend to use the various kinds of medical knowledge available to us to benefit others. The role of this high and altruistic intentionality has been central to medical practice from the days of Hippocrates.

One of the most controversial developments in the contemporary health care system concerns the degree to which health care can be considered a private market commodity. Private health care enterprises, such as Health Maintenance Organizations (HMOs) and privately owned hospitals, compete with non-profit hospitals and public hospitals. Physicians who work for HMOs can be thought of as employees who work regular hours for salaries, and some HMOs are owned by physician groups. The argument in favor of this type of system includes the claim that the "profit motive" is an incentive to provide high quality service at a reasonable price. Whether or not this claim is true, some physicians who work for private medical corporations become dissatisfied with the structure of their work because it conflicts with the altruistic intentions with which they entered medicine.

A physician on staff at Memorial Hospital, Dr. Molly Noonan, was talking with her colleagues one afternoon over coffee about what it was like working for an HMO. A resident asked her if she liked working regular hours.

"Well, at first, of course I did. It was my first job after my residency, which, as you know, is nothing if not irregular and exhausting. But after a while certain things about the job seemed wrong to me."

"For example?"

"If I left the office every day at five, I'd often have to cut short the time I like to spend with patients. Talking to patients is a part of good medicine, especially for a family practitioner. I felt as if I had to put my patients in slots in order to leave on time, which the HMO encouraged. Another problem was that I was under pressure to encourage my patients to undergo procedures, since that's where the money's at. Even if a patient has insurance, I don't think it's appropriate to recommend procedures that are unnecessary. At any rate, that decision wasn't entirely my own and the patient's."

"But a lot of patients feel like they're getting better care if they are referred to a specialist."

"But we shouldn't encourage those beliefs. And certainly such decisions shouldn't be made under administrative pressure. And just from a personal point of view, the physician working for an HMO is essentially working in isolation from everyone else. Here at Memorial we work in teams. At the HMO I worked at I could expect that every morning when I came into the office I'd have 20 phone calls to answer. I think the most distressing part of the job was feeling like I was an employee rather than a doctor. I couldn't focus on the needs of the patient. I also had to respond to the company's economic priorities."

"But don't you think that's happening here, too?"

"Sure. The competitive strategy is putting Memorial in a position of having to compete with private corporations, and public hospitals like County are really in trouble. It doesn't follow that for-profit medicine is the best medicine."

What do you think about Dr. Noonan's claim that for-profit medicine may not be the best medicine? Is for-profit medicine the "wave of the future", and if so will it distort or buttress the traditional altruistic intentions of health care professionals?

But reasoning and intentions must work reciprocally. The lead must be taken by knowledge and reasoning. All the best intentions in the world will not bring about good medical practice. So Aquinas puts prudence much more in the intellectual aspect of human behavior. We have to use our mind to regularly bend our will and desires to proper action.[20] The proper use of our intellect in practical maters involves the exercise of prudential counsel. Prudential judgment is a careful and judicious discerning. The constant demand for active use of knowledge in key medical decisions forces the constant use of a type of knowledge rather peculiar to medicine.[21]

But this particular kind of knowledge operates in its own way precisely because we are guided or even forced by our desires and intentions to not be content with merely abstract knowledge and speculation. Rather the task is to have particular principles which can be applied to particular cases.[22] Priorities must be set as to what can be accomplished in a case here and now. Our zeal and eagerness may sharpen our critical awareness, but it might also be obscured or blunted by haste.

Aquinas concludes that our powerful appetites and desires must be controlled and guided by a proper prudential ordering. With prudence remaining the central virtue, our choices and decisions are ethically enhanced by the practice of the virtue of justice. Courage or fortitude must regulate our aggressive drives; our concupiscible powers must be regulated by temperance.[23] The addition of the careful study of the habitual nature of these cardinal virtues enriches the Platonic–Aristotelian tradition in which they are rooted and provides us with a good deal of practical material for application to the contemporary situation of the practice of clinical medical ethics.

4

SCOTTISH MORAL SENSE

The Aristotelian–Platonic tradition of scholastic philosophy which has Thomas Aquinas as its central figure had an extremely long life. While it went through various stages often involving intense internal controversy it was still the basic type of philosophy taught in European universities into the 1700s. Partly because the tradition had too much mixed philosophy with theology, partly because too many primarily verbal disputes arose but mainly because the Aristotelian physics embedded in the system could not deal with the new findings in physics the Enlightenment philosophers searched for new approaches to perennial philosophical questions. In Scotland there was a very strong turn to the writings of Isaac Newton. His mastery of physics and the discovery of what were taken to be universal laws so different from the Aristotelian explanations seemed to be a key to the understanding of all reality.

This time of world colonization and the beginnings of the industrial revolution also posed a new set of ethical questions as the older settled social orders moved into a period of challenge and expansion. A number of Scottish thinkers became much involved in presenting programs to fit the new circumstances. In this they relied very heavily on the Newtonian approach. In Scotland there was a certain very pragmatic reason why this made a good deal of sense. The Scottish universities were thriving at this time. They had a set of strong curricular requirements. A student would be expected to pursue courses, for instance, in literature, mathematics, physics and philosophy. The physics would be Newtonian physics. Just as the physics part of the curriculum had been recently revised to bring it into line with the new science, so the philosophy parts of the curriculum were to undergo radical revision. This was especially true of two key parts of the philosophy program, epistemology and ethics. Epistemology is the study of the ways in which we perceive and know different aspects of the world around us. Newton's stress on the importance of empirical study forced a prioritizing in this area of sense and perceptual knowledge over the kind of abstract intellectualized speculation common to the scholastic tradition.

Needed was a more direct and simple way to deal with and process immediate information and evidence. So there developed a number of theories of knowledge which made sense knowledge or sensation primary. All of these theories also wanted to as much as possible reduce all knowledge to sense knowledge. This because even highly complex knowledge would be seen to be made up of quite simple and immediately accessible elements.

This epistemological revolution carried on immediatey into ethics. If sense knowledge is privileged in such a way as to directly and infallibly guide us to the reality of the physical world, then perhaps there is also a kind of moral sense which can directly cut through the complexities of the ethical realm. An ambiguity here will haunt this approach. There are at least two senses of sensing being used. One is the epistemological sense which refers to the experience of the five basic external senses. The other refers more to the emotive factor in ethical knowledge and decision making. So while the moral sense is modeled on the pattern of the workings of external sensation, it is really a strong introduction of emotive factors into ethics. The attempt is made, however, to keep these emotive factors as simple as possible. Just as physical sensation is clear, direct and uncluttered, so must moral sense simply and directly solve even the most complex of ethical dilemmas.

In Scotland the stress on the empirical aspects of Newton's work strongly tended to miss the enormous amount of quite abstract mathematical theory involved. Rather it was presumed that you could move from sense empirical knowledge quite directly to the abstract principles of physics, the most universal of them being the pushings and pullings embedded in the laws of universal gravitation. Because there was such a close connection between empirical sensation and these laws, the laws were considered to be ingrained right into matter itself. One could then in a way directly perceive these laws in experience of sensation.

This unity of immediate perception and abstract law or principle was most useful for the revolution in ethics. Morality and ethics is always a matter of a considerable number of rules, regulations and principles. Perhaps a way might be found to make these principles clear, simple, direct and easily perceived. This would also nicely fit with our basic experience of ethics, as it seems the case that every person has the simple and direct ability to understand and act ethically. This stress on the role and importance of individual ethical judgment will get a very strong hearing in the infant United States of America. Many of the university and high school (a Scottish term) curricula at this time in the young republic were based on the Scottish model as many of the teachers and professors came from there.[1]

The first Scottish philosopher to rigidly develop a theory of moral sense was Francis Hutcheson. While at first sight his use of Newtonianism may seem rather naive, the simplicity of his approach and its immediate applicability to practical situations make it still appealing and useful. Hutcheson thought that since Newton had shown that all of physical reality was rooted in the gravitational principles of attraction and repulsion so ethical reality has only two basically opposing principles, benevolence and self-interest. Just as in Newtonian physics the basic force is really gravitational attraction and repulsion is really a smaller example of this larger force at work, so for Hutcheson benevolence is the universal ethical principle and force with self-interest just an example of this force not working at its best.[2]

Apart from the naive transfer of Newtonian principles to the ethical sphere, Hutcheson remains a very important philosophical figure not only for the work he did in ethics but also for his theories of aesthetics. The two come together in a preliminary understanding of his approach to moral sense ethics. Just as we speak of certain people having a more highly developed aesthetic sense than others, so we might note that some people are more morally sensitive than others. To stay for a moment with the aesthetic sense, there does seem to be a certain inborn ability to create and appreciate art. But there are clearly many more people who can enjoy and appreciate art than those who can create it.

One of the areas of controversy in the practice of clinical medical ethics has to do with who should be the main expert in the field. Some maintain that only the practicing physician should be doing medical ethics at all as this is the only individual who really knows what is going on in the situation well enough to really understand. Also, since the physician is the one who ultimately must make the decision, all ethics should be in the physician's hands.

Others say that ethics must be a carefully learned discipline. It is so complicated and abstract that only the most expert person preferably trained at the doctorate level in philosophical ethics should attempt it.

Perhaps Hutcheson's assimilation of aesthetics to ethics can help us here. It is quite clear that some people have a natural aptitude to be physicians and others do not. That aptitude is rather like the sort of skill possessed by an artist. This because the practice of medicine is very much the practice of an art or skill. One learns it by doing it and one gets better at it by constantly staying in practice. But a drawback of this for both the artist and the physician is that it is rare indeed that an artist or a physician is a very good creative individual outside of the range of their specialty. Rarely do we find a painter who is also a good writer, or a musician who is also a fine sculptor. The skilled surgeon is rarely a good pediatrician; the expert cardiologist a fine oncologist. Creativity, artistic or medical is limited.

But the critical appreciation of both art and medicine can be much more broad. It is not unusual for a painter to enjoy music, for a cardiologist to appreciate the work of a fine surgeon. Ethics is more like this kind of critical appreciative sense. But even more so in that everyone to some degree or other has this sense whereas not everyone seems to have an aesthetically critical sense. Or even if it is true that everyone has some aesthetic sense, it seems to be more minimal in a large number of people than an ethical sense. Both the aesthetic and ethical sense need a good deal of training and development in order to become sharp and accurate.

Professional artists as well as professional philosopher–ethicists tend to be loners. They are quite aware of their own unique gifts and are rather jealous in the defense of them. Their very claim to fame or at least job security often depends on the uniqueness of their individual contribution. Physicians must work as part of a team. They learn medicine in the last years of medical school by close work with the team of professors and residents. The residency years themselves are a severe test of team adaptation and skills. Even when it comes to specialties and sub-specialties the members of the particular service must work creatively and harmoniously together.

So medical creativity is like the actively creative artistic sense. Since ethics is like the more passive aesthetic sense, the practicing clinical medical ethicist must initially play a more passive role. But the ethicist must be an integral part of the medical team. In a certain sense abstract theoretical ethics is not really ethics at all as the acid proof as to whether an ethical theory is correct or not is if it really works in real concrete situations.

As there are levels of active creative aesthetic and medical sense, so there are levels of more passive aesthetic and ethical sense. Certain individuals have more of a knack for one or the other. The physician just does not have time in the course of studies or practice to develop in detail the ethical skills now needed particularly when cases become increasingly complex and difficult in today's expanding world of medical and social realities. A well trained clinical medical ethicist can be of great help. But the ethicist and the physician must know that for some time the ethicist must be more critically passive in order to assess the moral dimensions of the situation. Then when judicious ethical advice is given the appreciative skills of the ethicist can combine with the creative skills of the physician in the communal practicing of medically and ethically sound medicine.

Ralph Watkins, a 75-year-old married man, was admitted to the intensive care unit of a university hospital in acute respiratory distress. He was anxious but fully alert and gasping for help. A retired laborer, Mr. Watkins had been suffering from a chronic pulmonary disease for the past fifteen years. For the past five years he had become progressively debilitated. Prior to admission he had been confined to his home and depended on his wife for the most basic care: without her assistance he could not dress or feed himself. He had been a fiercely independent man and still enjoyed ordering people around. His wife and married son were totally devoted to him.

The diagnosis was bilaterial pneumonia, and Mr. Watkins was given antibiotics and put on a mechanical respirator with supplemental oxygen. Within two weeks the pneumonia was largely cleared and Sarah Radburn, his physician, began attempts to wean him from the respirator. Unfortunately, he had become "respirator-dependent" as a result of a combination of poor nutrition, possible new damage to his lungs, weakened respiratory muscles, and fear of breathing on his own. Despite a slow, cautious approach with much reassurance, the weaning attempts repeatedly failed. Mr. Watkins, short of breath and terrified, would demand to be placed back on the respirator.

Dr. Radburn rated the ultimate chance for successful weaning as "maybe 20 per cent." The patient became more and more discouraged with his lack of progress and the frequent painful medical procedures. After three weeks of unsuccessful efforts, Mr. Watkins refused to cooperate with further attempts at weaning. His wife and son became concerned that he had given up the "will to live." They begged the medical staff to "do something to save him." Although he had become less communicative, he remained alert and aware and, in the opinion of the staff, was fully competent. He told Dr. Radburn he wanted the respirator disconnected. "I want to die," he said.

Dr. Jones, the ethicist at the hospital, had been brought in for a consult when Mr. Watkins first started demanding to be placed back on the respirator. That was fortunate, since Dr. Jones needed to observe the situation as it developed over the three-week process. He suggested to Dr. Radburn that she shouldn't jump to any conclusions, since she had to weigh several different values: the patient's autonomy, his suffering, the family's feelings and the medical imperative of beneficence.

He pointed out that several resources had not yet been tried, such as a psychiatric consult, social work services and a community health center that provided home support for chronically ill patients. He also suggested a conference with everyone involved to explain the law to the family. In their state, the law prohibits shutting off the respirator until the patient is weaned, which would mean that Mr. Watkins would be on a respirator until he either lost all cortical function or relaxed enough to permit weaning.

In the end, Mr. Watkins was successfully weaned and returned home with nursing and psychotherapeutic services provided by the community health program. Can you think of any other creative responses that Dr. Jones and the medical team might have brought to this situation?

A new and dramatic development for the role of the clinical medical ethicist has, however, recently taken place. As rounding clinical medical ethicists have become more known and accepted in hospital settings demands have been made on them to play not only an advisory role but also to be active participants in key critical decisions. Many hospitals as a result now have ethical consult services. These services can be called in on consult just as other medical consult services. A number of ethicists are on call and can be reached by beeper. This consult may be so formal as to require that the ethicist document and sign in the patient's chart. This development moves the ethicist from the role of more passive critical team member to creative ethicist. Since the majority of the cases which require such a formal consult are indeed very tough and complex ones, a good deal of ethical creativity is demanded. Since the answers are not clear and simple a creative ethical solution must be found for this unique case. Here clearly the ethicist is assuming more the stance of the creative physician or artist. So there is a growing area in which, as a member of the medical team, the clinical ethicist makes a directly positive contribution. It is very important to be aware of the changing dynamics and modalities of the types of medicine and ethics being practiced by different members of the team in different times and circumstances.

It was 1 a.m. when a young man came into the emergency room of Memorial Hospital with severe abdominal pain. He was triaged to the surgery side with a surgery intern and a family practice intern working that night. The surgery intern began taking the history. The patient denied any past medical history or being in any "high-risk" group. Meanwhile, the patient vomited blood and vomitus all over the surgery intern during the physical exam.

While this was happening, the family practice intern was looking through the old chart and saw the patient had previously tested HIV+ and was taking AZT. The family practice intern told the surgery intern this while he was cleaning up the mess. The surgery intern was furious that the patient had lied to him and had put him at risk, and he refused to have anything more to do with the patient.

The family practice intern called in the ethicist on call to discuss with them the moral and legal situation. When Dr. Jones arrived a couple of minutes later, he saw immediately that the two interns had somewhat different moral perspectives. The surgeon saw his role not as a primary care giver (which may include cleaning up a mess), but as a skilled practitioner who was there to do his job as well and as quickly as possible. He also faced greater risks than the family practice intern, who would not have to come into contact with the patient's blood during an operation.

The family practice intern, on the other hand, did see himself as primary care giver, and considered anything short of seeing this patient through this crisis as abandonment. Perhaps because he also did not see himself as at as great a risk as the surgical intern for contracting HIV, he had sufficient distance from personal feelings (including fear) to sympathize with the patient's desire to protect his privacy. Hence, the family practice intern was less offended by the patient's lying about his HIV status.

The ethicist explained to the surgeon that in the ER he was obligated by law to try to stabilize the patient. But in order to discuss some of the moral and situational issues mentioned above, the ethicist arranged to meet with both interns later that day. The surgery intern was persuaded to help stabilize the patient.

Because everyone has some at least minimal aesthetic and more ethical sense, there is a need to explain the complexities of medicine and ethics to other people, especially to the patient and the patient's family. Here Hutcheson can again help. He thinks that the basic principles of both aesthetics and ethics are really quite simple so that anyone can understand them. The individuals who are skilled in the complexities only really have that skill by proving that they can again translate it back into simple language and concepts for the average person.

One of the characteristics of both the aesthetic and ethical senses is its simplicity. It is very hard to explain just why ultimately something is beautiful or good. It just is. So the creative physician and the skilled ethicist must be looking for simplicity. They should be looking for uniformity in variety.[3]

This seems to ring quite true in the practice of medicine and ethics. So much of it is done by analogy with other like cases. When similarities appear it is of great help in the solution of a case. Hutcheson also says that there is a certain amount of self-interest or utility involved in the discovery of these similarities. A few laws or principles are more easy to remember. Reduction to simple terms makes the basic practice of virtue more easy.[4] Certainly in the stress and strain of clinical medicine it is helpful to have some basic principles to which one can rather directly go. But it must always be kept in mind that these principles are only so strong as the many years of training that make them. Simplicity does not come easy.

But Hutcheson is quite concerned that we do not place a great deal of stress on the intellectual content of these principles. Rather he points out that our actions are much more motivated by feelings and emotions than by clear thought patterns. By this he means to say that we have to have some sort of motivation in order to be properly involved in creative activity.[5] This would be especially true in the case of any activity with a clear ethical dimension.

The medical profession has always been one which puts a very strong stress on high ideals. One simply must be a very dedicated person to put up day after day, year after year with the demands and stresses of the profession. There must be the ever present commitment to excellence. And Hutcheson notes that this is precisely his central moral sense of benevolence. It is clear to both insiders and outsiders of the practice of medicine that it is a passionate affair. In fact any attempt by the profession or by individual practitioners to portray medicine as a remote and coldly abstract discipline is met by disapproval both from within and without medicine.

Clearly there is a strong academic and intellectual element. But that aspect is in service of the more passionate commitment, not the other way round.[6] In medical terms this means that knowledge is not to be pursued for its own sake but only because we so strongly desire to bring about the cure and ease of the patient that we study and research every possible avenue. This can become problematic in academic medicine where the quest for knowledge or the need to build up personal prestige or academic status can be a strong lure towards putting the intellectual factor first and the strong drive to heal the patient second. This is most especially true when it comes to the area of experimental medicine.

There are a number of reasons why the problem becomes so acute here. The formulation of a protocol often really is not so concerned with patient health as with proving the effectiveness of a particular drug or therapy. Patient health is not disconnected from this kind of proof, but what is crucial is the setting of priorities. It is too easy to slip into research as the primary goal and to lose sight of the very purpose of the research itself. A recollection on the part of researchers that in all their procedures it is people they are trying to help will be of considerable use in keeping priorities straight.

A second problem with research medicine is the use of the double blind. Even though patient consent is obtained and as a result the patients know that they may just be getting a placebo, there is a kind of hope which the patients hold out for cure or amelioration even though the situation may be rather bleak or hopeless. Fascination and concentration on the part of both the research physician and the patients with the technical aspects of the research procedures can shift priorities from cure and care to more remote and abstract academic possibilities. The research physician must always remain a doctor who is driven to do everything possible to care for this research subject patient.

When medical research first began on the AIDS-effective drug

AZT, there were no other effective treatments. Hence, they had to use a placebo as a control. Since AIDS is so far incurable and, as far as we can tell, fatal, there were plenty of volunteers for the experiments. About half the subjects, however, received the placebo.

At that time (1986), FDA regulations were very strict and methodologically adequate tests were required before AZT coud be put on the market. That meant that sufficient trials were required to establish statistical significance. The physicians on the research teams were often the primary physicians for the subjects.

Before a high level of statistical significance was achieved, however, it was clear that AZT had some effect in ameliorating the symptoms of certain AIDS-related diseases. The physicians had to decide whether or not to continue the experiment. In this case they stopped the double-blind trials, offered AZT to all the subjects who wanted it, and continued to follow their progress. The personal care of the subjects in this series of trials took priority over the need to satisfy strict methodological criteria.

One of the ways of making clear what really are our aims in the practice of any sound ethics, including medical ethics, is to make sure that even though we are rightly under the strong influence of a passion or desire we concentrate on the object of that desire not on the desire or passion in itself. Hutcheson here is much influenced by another important moral sense theorist, Joseph Butler.[7] But our emotions remain our guides in making sure that we are concentrating on the proper object.[8] Certain emotions are better than others as we attempt to use them to keep our aims clear. As long as these emotions are more clearly suffused with a sense of altruism the better chance they have of helping us to be objective. But Hutcheson is very strong on this kind of emotive experience. He is convinced that we really do feel quite strongly when we are acting more ethically correctly than when we are not.[9] This is a good guide then to keep us objective. Rather clearly when we do not feel right about what we are doing, objectivity can quickly go. If we get to the situation of not really feeling good about our actions in a particular case, that is certainly a good indication that an ethical consult should be called to help with the restoration of objectivity.

There is a serious problem, however, with the adapting of such an emotive ethic with such a stress on benevolence. Because this kind of ethic is so concerned to do the best possible in any given situation, it can overlook larger questions of justice. This has a particular bite in the medical field. In many ways medical ethics is out of step with larger ethical issues in American life. The country takes great pride in its sense of liberty and justice for all. We tend to take a large overview of all of the people and try to make sure that everyone as much as possible has an equal opportunity to achieve the highest goals of which they are capable. This clearly does not always work, but the ideal remains. There is a stress on individuals as part of larger groups. Justice for all means making sure that each and every member of the group has equal opportunity.

Medicine operates in a different way. Patients are people who already to some degree or other have their opportunities curtailed. Physicians cannot deal with them as equals. Rather the physician is in an authority position because of greater expertise and access to curative measures. Each patient must not be be considered to be a part of a larger democratic whole but as a special individual case often in desperate need of help. So benevolence and a strong altruistic moral sense work well in medicine but a sense of justice for all is not very operative.

In this time of limitations on health care because of rising costs and growing populations, the individual practitioner is not in a strong position to have a good and clear overall view of the larger needs of the general population. But people outside of medicine, including lawmakers, also do not have a good perspective on the situation as they do not understand the demands of medicine itself. Some kind of stronger working relationship is needed so that the benevolence of medicine can be better exercised in a framework of justice for all.

Mr. Avery, a 70-year-old man living on social security and with no insurance other than Medicare, felt like he had a bad case of indigestion. But when it didn't pass, he called up his daughter, who lives two blocks away. When she arrived at his house, she saw immediately that he was having a heart attack. She drove him to the nearest hospital, which is a proprietary facility.

They admitted Mr. Avery to the emergency room, while his daughter started filling out forms at the admitting desk. The person at the admitting desk asked her if her father had insurance:

"No, except for Medicare."

"Does he have any savings or income to pay for his care?"

"No, he lives on social security, and I'm unemployed right now. So I don't have any insurance that would cover him."

The clerk told her that they would have to transfer Mr. Avery to a public hospital as soon as he was stabilized, because they could not guarantee that Medicare would pay for his care under the DRG Prospective Payment System.

In fact, however, this hospital had set up a policy for transferring patients who could not pay their bills, and that policy penalized physicians for keeping such patients. The physician in charge of Mr. Avery was so anxious to avoid a penalty that he certified Mr. Avery was stable when he was not. By the time Mr. Avery arrived at the county hospital, he had had a cardiac arrest and was dead on arrival.

It is important to keep in mind that cost containment initiatives, like the DRG PPS can affect decisions made at the bedside with sometimes disastrous results.

Hutcheson makes a first start at this by noting that there is a difference between motivating and justifying reasons. Motivating reasons are very closely tied to our original affections or emotions. These are the sort of experiences which get us to act at all ethically. In medical terms these would be the basic inner drives which lead us first to pursue and then to continue the practice of medicine. Justifying reasons are more closely connected to the moral sense as such. They would be ways in which to understand the workings of the moral sense. We might, for instance, be able to reason about means to ends.[10] This would correspond to the working through of detail so essential in medical practice.

But because Hutcheson places ethics so securely in the inner sense of morality which we all have any rational study of ethics is highly problematic. The stress on inner emotive drives is well taken and much needed in our time, but there is clearly here an over-stress. The only way that Hutcheson can consistently work his way out of this is to appeal to a range of emotive experience which can foster and bolster the moral sense. So there is an appeal to a sense of honor, shame, sympathy, veracity, courtesy and more.[11]

This is a move back into the virtue tradition of ethics inasmuch as these kinds of ethical senses are the ones which we would find in the situations of human interaction which Aristotle made the central genesis of ethical behavior and whose habitual character Aquinas stressed. Hutcheson tries to keep these virtues securely anchored in his theory of benevolent moral sensism by ranking the virtues somewhat. The most excellent virtues are kind affections, beneficent purposes and the love of moral excellence. A lower class of virtues includes friendship, general courtesy deportment.[12] While this is fashioned in this way so as to stress the central function of benevolence, there is an application to medical practice in that the need to work out in practice the basically simple benevolent drives that are operative in medicine involves the constant working with colleagues in which a great number of what Hutcheson calls the lower class of virtues are constantly put to the test. In the pressure of working to solve a patient's problem we may very well practice a very good ethics of the physician–patient relationship while at the same time be violating all sorts of ethics in our dealings with colleagues and subordinates. A really just ethical approach will involve all the parties to the decisions and actions.

Mrs. Billings had undergone a radical mastectomy at John Sealy Hospital in Texas, and was recuperating from the operation. When women have mastectomies they customarily are provided with a special gown that opens from the front in a way that protects their privacy during post-operative examinations. But in Mrs. Billings' case, the nurse, Ms. Roland, had not been able to locate the special gown, and had to give her a standard gown.

When Dr. Smith, her surgeon, saw that she did not have the special gown, he furiously called the nurse: "Roland, bring in the proper gown immediately". When the nurse arrived, Dr. Smith started screaming at Ms. Roland: "You know Mrs. Billings should have been given this gown in the first place, don't you?"

"Yes, but . . . "

"I don't want to hear any excuses! If you can't do your job properly, don't do it at all!"

He grabbed the old gown and threw it on the floor. He continued his tirade, in front of Mrs. Billings, for several more minutes. Then he dismissed Ms. Roland, who appeared shaken and extremely embarrassed.

Mrs. Billings was so disturbed by Dr. Smith's public display of anger that she called a medical humanities professor associated with John Sealy, whom she had met several times. Mrs. Billings was very upset about the arrogance and lack of courtesy with which Dr. Smith had handled the situation, and needed to talk with someone about it.

There was nothing wrong with Dr. Smith's clinical relationship with Mrs. Billings up to that point. Indeed, he had always been very sensitive to the feelings of his patients. Nonetheless, his relationship with the nursing staff had a disturbing impact on his patient's hospital experience, as well as on the nurse's sense of self-respect.

Another Scottish philosopher, David Hume, worked much more on the notion of justice in ethics. He wanted to ground ethics not solely in the subjective inner personal sense of altruistic benevolence but rather in a balance between self-interest and a more limited benevolence. There is, however, an appeal to a sort of a guiding sense, in this case a sense of sympathy.[13] But sympathy is a through and through social sense. Our proximity to each other and the close interactions which we have with each other demand that we act ethically toward each other. Sympathy is not so much directed to individual persons but to the more general welfare of social groups. The virtues which are practiced in social groups are naturally based on the need to make the group work harmoniously. Virtue takes on something of an artificial character when social conventions of a particular time or place dictate to a great extent how the natural sympathetic sense is in detail played out.[14]

Crucial to Hume's approach is that we take a sort of spectator view of morality. This means that the notion of sympathy is not so much an interiorly felt or experienced emotion as an observation on what is actually the best kind of empirically noted human behavior. Sympathy would be the general binding force in human affairs. A sense of duty would be secondary to sympathy as a first place position for duty would tend to make ethics too personal and emotive.[15] Certain other second place ethical emotions such as pride or love would lead to virtue. Others such as humility or hatred would lead to vice.[16] The practice of virtuous action would be a sign of a good character. We would be able to observe that people of good character would tend to practice virtues such as prudence, temperance, frugality, industry, assiduity, enterprise, dexterity, generosity and humanity.[17] We can note that this is pretty much a description of the proper English or Scottish gentleman of the day.

Hume has loomed large as a much more important philosophical figure than Hutcheson. The reason is, that while he uses the language of emotion and virtue, the whole way of doing philosophy is changed by Hume. There is little personal involvement, but rather a coldly empirical examination of the situation as we find it. It is vital that we be impartial spectators at the scene. Any account of ethics is at one or two removes from the actual engagement in ethics. The study of the structures of ethics is important, not ethical activity itself. From such a study one can get very little guidance or direction as to what just precisely ought to be done in resolving the complexities of an ethical dilemma.

Hume's influence has been massive in the subsequent development of Anglo-American ethics. Many professional philosophical ethicists sneer at those of us who practice applied ethics in such fields as medicine or business. It is considered soft or second rate philosophy and should not be trusted or taken seriously. Even if philosophy is to concern itself with practical questions, its functions should be quite severely restricted to the analysis of the types of logic and argumentation going on in applied ethics. On this model a rounding clinical medical ethicist's primary job would be to provide clarification of the often tangled logic of the clinical situation. The ethicist would rarely give any actual advice and even if this did occur the advice should not be taken too seriously. The ethicist rather would be more of a spectator to the process than an integral member of the clinical team.

There are also in Hume some rather strong strains of utilitarianism. The disinterested observer would note what appears to be working best for the greatest number of people. This kind of ethic might work rather well for social questions affecting the health care professions, but it does not lend itself well to problems of individual patient care.

The next figure we would like to consider is Adam Smith. He has an enormous reputation as the chief theorist of the kind of capitalist economy practiced basically throughout the free world. But he is also a most important moral theorist. He shares with Hume the use of a spectator. But this spectator is not so much disinterested as creative. This is seen very clearly in his economic theory where one of the deepest reasons given for our confident use of a free market system is that there is an "invisible hand" which is at work making a larger sense of the multiple give and take of free trade.[18] All we have to do is to keep playing hard with the bits and pieces of the economic system and the larger pattern will emerge and create ever new market opportunities. While this may seem naive a few centuries of its practice have shown that it seems to be far and away the best approach.

What is most interesting and revolutionary about Smith's economic theory is that for the invisible hand to creatively work well an individual engaged in trying to make a profit cannot primarily concentrate on trying to maximize individual advantage.

Rather you have to put first the advantage of the other person. If, for instance, you can market a product of such a quality for such a price as it is your buyer's advantage to purchase it, then you will get the profit from this. So there is a kind of radically pragmatic altruism built into this type of economics.

The application to medical practice is clear and direct. Doctors remain in this country some of the purest practitioners of Smithian economics. They are in business by and large for themselves. The rise of Health Maintenance Organizations and Preferred Provider Groups is viewed with suspicion. But any physician who aims first and foremost primarily at making money will not long be very good in the practice of medicine. Even the money side of medicine must somehow look first not to the good of the doctor but to the good of the patient. A physician who does not put the patient financially first is in considerable danger of losing reputation and practice.

On December 5, 1986, Rosa R. presented to the emergency room at DeTar Hospital in Victoria, Texas. She was pregnant, had received no prenatal care, and reported that her membranes had ruptured spontaneously at 3.15 p.m.

Upon initial examination there was vaginal discharge, wetness and leakage, but membranes were intact, and fluid was still palpable in front of the fetus' head. Mrs. R.'s blood pressure was 210/130 mm Hg. She was having moderate 60-second uterine contractions every three minutes that had begun at 7 a.m. Her cervix was 2–3 cm dilated and 60–70 per cent effaced; and a nitrazine test was positive. She was at or near term by dates and the fetal head was ballottable.

The summoning nurse reported that she asked Dr. B. by telephone to examine Mrs. R. at 4.15 p.m., and that he told her to arrange for Mrs. R. to be transferred to John Sealy Hospital, about 160 miles away.

Dr. B. examined the patient about 4.30 p.m., and contacted a physician at Sealy Hospital, who accepted the transfer and suggested that magnesium sulfate be given. Dr. B. ordered magnesium sulfate and bed rest for hypertension and present preeclampsia and ordered the transfer. He signed a transfer certificate required by the Department of Health and Human Services, stating that he believed the transfer's benefits outweighed the risks. He did not order any special medication or life-support equipment for Mrs. R.'s trip to Sealy Hospital.

About 30 miles from Victoria, Mrs. R. gave birth to a healthy boy, and insisted she wanted to go back home. Dr. B. refused to assume continued responsibility for her treatment, but he agreed to allow another physician to examine her when she returned to DeTar.

DeTar is a for-profit health care facility, and John Sealy hospital is the closest public hospital in that part of Texas. Mrs. R. is on Welfare, and Medicaid in Texas is very inadequate. Dr. B. considered the risks of treating her to outweigh the benefits, he claimed at his court hearing. While this may be true, the standard of care for a woman in active labor would prohibit transfer to a hospital 160 miles away. Do you think her poverty might have influenced the doctor's judgment in this case? Who should estimate risks and burdens when financial considerations must enter into the calculation?

But the concern for others which Smith had proposed in economics has an even stronger place in his theory of ethics. There is a strong use of the sympathy factor but it is combined by Smith with both subjective and objective perspectives. Sympathy remains the root of morals but only when in community we take on the other person's point of view.[19] In order to do this we must be something also of a disinterested spectator. This distinteretedness is achieved by objectifying our own subjective moral perspective. When we take on another person's moral point of view, just as when we work to achieve the economic advantage of the other person, an invisible hand works to bring about the best ethical outcome. There is a very strong pragmatism here in that the ultimate reason why both economics and ethics are right is because they work so well. We will be wanting to examine carefully some other versions of pragmatism in the next chapter.

Before we go on to some other aspects of Smith's ethics, consider for a moment the use of the disinterested observer and the concern for other's motives in the clinical practice of medicine. Certainly one of the most commonly used arguments on the part of physicians takes the form of putting one's self in the patient's shoes. Many times one hears physicians saying that if they were in the patient's position they would or would not like certain procedures done. One especially seems to hear this a good deal from residents. Perhaps it is because for the first time they are taking actual responsibility for their own decisions and so they fall back to this rather simple approach. This is a very tricky move. It is first of all in its naive form highly deceptive. I cannot put myself in the other person's position, because I am in my own position and not in that of the other person. As a result what may appear to be a highly objective argument is in fact subjective. And it is badly subjective in that one may believe that an objective move has really been made.

Smith has a saving element here. He notes that you have to take on the other person's point of view in a disinterested way. That is the force of noting that morality and the taking on the other's view is only to be done in the context of the community in which both parties are working. Since the medical team is regularly a large one, this might suggest that in trying to take on the point of view of the patient I might have to consider what all of the members of the team think might be the patient's point of view. This would certainly allow for a good deal of pragmatic objectivity in the working out of ethical decisions.

Mrs. Rose Smith is a 72-year-old black woman admitted to the geriatric medicine service with a large pelvic mass. She is a very spry old lady and is very much interested in having her way and maintaining control over what happens to her in the hospital. She is quite pleasant, and greets her doctors in the morning "Good morning, how are you doing this morning?" When the doctors reply "How are you doing Mrs. Smith?", she always replies "I'm doing just fine." The problem is that medically she isn't doing just fine. She has a rather large mass in her belly and she has not eaten well in months. Her nutritional status is very poor, making her a poor surgical candidate. The mass in her belly is probably making her feel full, and she has no desire to eat. She steadfastly refuses to have a feeding tube placed, stating that she doesn't "want that thing put up my nose." In addition, Mrs. Smith is an eccentric lady. At one point she carefully wrapped up a plate of food in tissue and placed it in a corner of her room, refusing to eat it and requesting that it not be moved for several days. A nurse finally threw it away when Mrs. Smith was not paying attention.

Thus the doctors have a problem. They are caring for an eccentric patient with a pelvic mass that needs to be taken out and the patient agrees. But she is a poor surgical candidate because of her nutritional status; it is not likely to improve because she will not or cannot eat. The "solution" to the problem – the feeding tube – is definitely refused by the patient. The question becomes: do the doctors force the patient to accept the feeding tube?

In a situation like this, it might be helpful to try to understand the motivational point of view of the patient. If you don't force your own conception of what ought to be done on the patient, you might open up lines of communication that will facilitate finding a way to persuade the patient to take the feeding tube, at least for a while. Can you imagine a conversation with this patient in which a treatment plan could be devised by everyone involved, but with primary attention focused on the patient's point of view?

The place of pragmatism in Smith's thought deserves more careful consideration. In many ways he developed a quite radical approach to philosophy and ethics which has a strongly contemporary ring. This because of his use of Newtonianism. Unlike many of the Newtonians of his day Smith did not think that Newton had once and for all solved all the problems of physics. Rather he thought that Newton had constructed a grand imaginative scheme of immense pragmatic use. Physics and philosophy begin in puzzlement and wonder at an unexplained set of objects or events. The role of imagination is crucial in the attempt to make connections.[20] Imagination is also seen as a sort of machine which puts together the various parts of things. (Our more biologically inclined age might see this more as a creative life force.) There is a strong recognition that this creative imagination has not solved all questions but provides for the time as good an explanation as possible. New times and new questions will require more imaginative solutions.

Ethics is often presented as a matter of right and wrong, but perhaps it should better be presented as a matter of better and best or worse and worst. This would particularly be true in the case of clinical medical ethics. We are confronted by a set of circumstances that make it difficult to decide just how best to proceed. The solution reached should not claim to be an ultimate final ethical solution for this and all like cases, but rather our best imaginative solution in the practical pragmatic situation. New clinical situations demand new creative ethical solutions. All ethics but especially clinical ethics should look always to the future not to the past.

Smith spells out his pragmatism by re-working in detail Hume's notion of sympathy. It is a really careful examination of the taking on of another person's point of view which is so central to Smith's ethics.

There are four sources of moral approbation. They hark back to Hutcheson's motivating reasons as Smith is concerned to anchor any objectivism in ethics in the kind of emotive subjectivism presented by his Scottish predecessor. The first of these sources, propriety, is sympathy with someone else's motives.[21] The second, is merit, which is sympathy with someone's gratitude. The third, which is a lesser consideration, is sympathy with the general rules of morality. In order to bring this into play the role of the disinterested spectator must be invoked. A final source of moral approbation is utility, but this is not central and is treated by Smith as something of an afterthought.[22]

The stress on interpersonal interaction and not on rules and utility makes Smith's approach very congenial to clinical medical ethics. It is vital that the physician practice propriety in trying to reach some undertanding of what might be the patient's motives in seeking and pursuing treatment. All too often the patient is seen as presenting with a particular problem or complaint and then is treated as a clinical example of a particular kind of medical situation outlined in the textbooks and current literature. Understanding and empathizing with motivational factors will move the whole physician-patient relationship into one of mutual respect and concern. The doctor will then be able to play the helping role which is so central to medicine at its best. We will then be doing the best kind of ethics that we can in the situation.

Such motivational factors can be of crucial importance in certain kinds of disease situations. It would be very important to know what caused a person who gets diagnosed as having a particular kind of cancer to seek treatment. Was it because of noted pain or bodily disfunction or was it because of a more general concern for health? A person who sought a check-up because of a practice of heavy smoking and a fear of consequences would be different perhaps in many ways from a person who felt severe chest pain and so sought help. One might be motivated to stop smoking, the other not at all. The same sort of scenario could be played out by cardiac and many other patients. The role of motivating factors in long term care patients such as many of them working with endocrinologists could well be critical.

Propriety might seem a rather strange name to give to such concern for others' motives, but it fits in well with a well-worn theme in medical ethics. Victorian medical ethics was very strong on the physician observing the proper proprieties. This would mean not only the rules of politeness but also a very discrete set of interpersonal relationships. This kind of reticence is still often at play in medical practice. It offers a support to the treating of the patient as a clinical specimen, not as another human being. But in this age of more openness moves should be made to take on the motivational point of view of the patient. Most patients will be quite pleased with this as they will find themselves being treated as real human beings in a relationship with another caring and competent helper. There are dangers here but the chances are high that the physician engaging in these kinds of interactions will find the practice of medicine to be the satisfying and supportive calling to which they best respond.

Dr. Jones was an idealistic first year resident who noticed that the surgical attending may have made a mistake in judgment.

Baby O., a blond-haired, blue-eyed, playful one-year-old had suffered a deep second degree burn to the left side of his face, both above and below the eye. Dr. Jones first felt pity, because he feared the child might be disfigured for life. Baby O. had been burned by accidental contact with a hot motorcycle muffler two weeks before, and needed a skin graft to aid the healing process.

Dr. Jones discussed the situation with Baby O.'s parents, and had felt much sympathy for them as well. He knew they were suffering a great deal.

When Baby O. was admitted to the general surgery service, the attending decided to use a split thickness skin graft to cover the wound. This surprised Dr. Jones. He had learned in medical school that a full thickness graft offers less skin contraction and a better cosmetic result than a split thickness graft, even though the latter has a somewhat higher "take rate". When Dr. Jones suggested to the attending that Baby O. might do better with a full thickness graft, the attending said, "Look, he'll need another operation when he gets older anyway."

Remembering the fear on the face of the parents, he persisted in trying to persuade the attending to rethink his decision. In the end, Baby O. received a full thickness graft, and recovered nicely. But the resident had taken a certain risk in challenging the attending's judgment.

After the operation, Baby O.'s parents expressed their gratefulness effusively. At first, Dr. Jones was uncomfortable with this show of emotion, but he did not discourage it. Two years later when he was chief resident and working under a great deal of pressure, Baby O.'s parents walked into his office with their child in tow and thanked him again. Baby O. had recovered very well indeed, and now Dr. Jones felt grateful that Baby O.'s parents held him in such high esteem.

Smith does use the term, merit, in a way in which we would not. But the aspect of ethics which he is trying to bring out is well worth consideration. Merit is sympathy with someone's gratitude. Smith has it in his system because this would stress very strongly the role of another person's emotions in the balance between objective and subjective. But in medical practice we regularly experience a great outpouring of gratitude to the physician on the part of patients and patients' families. Often the gratitude is not commensurate with the care and help being provided, but patients are so grateful in a time of need that they must express their feelings. Rather than repressing or ignoring these feelings, physicians will do well to integrate them into practice. They provide a rich source for motivation for cure and care. Also they form a strong base for an enduring physician-patient relationship of mutual support. Strong emotions on both sides run in these relationships. They are the life blood of the ethics involved. Smith is quite right to see these emotions as the primary foundation of ethics.

The clinical ethical experience also shows the secondary place Smith assigns to the use of general rules and principles of utility. The more there is a direct appeal to these last two the more there is the chance that the clinical encounter will be stiff and inhuman. Nobody quite fits into any general rule and no one should be treated primarily in terms of the general usage that they have in keeping going a personal practice or medical center operation. Motivating emotions will keep us close to the really central supportive functions and goals of medicine. While there is a little idealism here, this is a good thing as medicine certainly is one of the most idealistic professions possible. An idealism at its best is often ethics at its best.

Sometimes rules and principles can't help us make tragic choices because the relevant principles themselves conflict. There are times when respect for rights conflicts with our disposition to prevent suffering. Consider a case such as the following: Bradley is the seven-year-old son of staunch Jehovah's Witnesses. One night, about 10 p.m., the family was in an auto accident. Everyone except Bradley suffered minor bruises and scratches. Bradley, however, is brought into the nearest hospital trauma unit, bleeding profusely.

He will need transfusion of blood and blood products, if he is to survive the night. The resident at the trauma unit has asked the parents to sign a consent form, authorizing the trauma team to begin the blood transfusions that Bradley needs to survive.

The parents refuse to sign the consent form, insisting that Bradley himself is unconscious. On the one hand, the physician is morally required to get consent for any procedure from either the patient or the patient's decision-making surrogates, who in this case are Bradley's parents. But the physician also has an obligation to save Bradley's life. How can we choose between conflicting moral principles?

In this situation, the physician must rely on her feelings of sympathy for Bradley. Bradley's parents' preferences, if followed, may result in his death. There is no time to get a court injunction, and even if there were, the moral problem would remain. Compassion and sympathy may move us to make the best *possible* choice, even when that choice violates an abstract rule.

Smith also is concerned to work his ethics into the grand tradition of virtue ethics which we have been exploring in this book. In this the notion of perfectionism plays a pragmatically central role. Guiding the ranking of the virtues is the ordered progression of the sources of moral approbation. The more a virtue is motivated by propriety the better it is. Merit motivates a slightly lesser group of virtues. Virtues practiced because they conform to rules or utility are not so ethically impressive. The virtues are divided into self-regarding and other-regarding. The single self-regarding virtue is prudence.[23] Propriety works here when we rid ourselves to some extent of selfish interests and take on the other person's point of view. The imaginative mechanism of the impartial spectator should guarantee this.

Justice and benevolence are other-regarding virtues. Justice is taken to be a rather minimalistic virtue. In exercising a sympathy with others the just person shares their feelings of resentment. This is a most telling and challenging point. American virtue and ethics is often built around justice as its radically basic and fundamental starting point. The American experience clearly did arise out of feelings of strong resentment against the British. As a result there is a danger that our ethics which so strongly stresses personal rights and freedom may be insensitive to social and altruistic concerns. We may have too minimalistic an ethic. This may be one of the reasons why medical ethics does not fit easily and well into the general American scene. It is interesting to see one of the pillars of capitalism, that other vital ingredient of Americanism, putting justice considerations rather at the bottom of his ethical scheme. But minimal as it is justice is an absolutely essential virtue for Smith.[24] Without it society would fall apart. This means that the rules of justice must be rigidly followed whereas the rules of prudence and benevolence are more broad. Since medical ethics is not so tied basically to justice, it is clear that in practice there is more latitude to the rules.

For Smith benevolence is the higher virtue. This involves a sharing of the feeling of altruism. So the virtues are ranked more along the lines of benevolence and prudence being better than justice. Hutcheson's influence is still strong in this transformed view of moral sense. But there is an ultimate Smithian virtue. This is the virtue of self-command.[25] This means a clear and emotively definite striving for what is ethically best and a dissatisfaction with anything else. Perfect knowledge of ethics may even stand in our way as it may make us complacent and keep us from the needed constant ethical effort. This out and out striving for perfection takes prudence, benevolence and justice to greater heights. In a different way this striving for perfection is rather like the Aristotelian and especially the Aquinistic recognition that in order for virtuous habits to function at all there must be constant effort to make them work at their best.

Par excellence (hence the use of these terms) medicine demands the skillful practice of medical and ethical perfection, so we would do well to take into account Smith's emotional call to immerse ourselves in the high calling of the profession.

A final figure that we should consider in this Scottish moral sense approach to ethics is Thomas Reid. He was somewhat critical of the too emotive approach of Hutcheson and Smith. Rather he uses emotive factors as cognitive elements themselves. Reid is concerned to note that belief plays a very large role in any kind of knowledge which we have.[26] But belief is essentially an act of commitment to certain perceived truths. It is basically an act of will.[27] We know what we decide to know. The more that we exercise our beliefs, the more we build up principles of knowledge and action. So knowledge is bound up with principles of practice. Applications to medicine and medical ethics are obvious.

Reid held that our belief commitment to a set of principles about the physical world led to our correct knowledge of that world. The same would hold in the ethical realm. We must be committed to a set of ethical principles which will help to illumine the ethical scene. Here are some of the salient features of these principles. We may be culpable in omitting what we ought to do as much in fact as in doing our duty. We ought to use the best means we can to be well informed of our duty by serious attention to moral instruction. We ought to prefer a greater good, though more distant, to a lesser good, a less evil to a greater evil. We ought to comply with the intentions of nature. We are not born for ourselves alone. In every case we ought to act that part toward another which we would judge right in that person to act towards us if we were in that person's circumstance and that person in ours.[28]

While clearly this is a rough and ready list, it does mirror rather well what in fact we in many cases do. We have a set of often very poorly articulated ethical principles. The reason that we have these principles at all according to Reid is that we have a voluntary belief commitment to them. We need and want a set of principles. The fact that there is such a voluntaristic aspect to this precludes the possibility of complete clarity in the principles. But here Reid has a strong difference from Smith. Smith held that we have principles of science and ethics, but he ties these principles to imagination rather than to belief. In this there is a danger of relativism because our imaginative creation of such principles can develop new and different principles as times and circumstances change.

Reid in his approach wants to have a more permanent place for these principles. He wants to maintain that our committed beliefs are not fundamentally misplaced. This is, of course, all still very much in the moral sensism frame of reference. We are simply dealing in Reid with a more voluntaristic type of moral sense. Yet there is something strongly here to be considered. The more that I want to be ethically correct, the more chance that I will act ethically. The less I want ethics, the less chance that I will act ethically. My desire to be ethical will lead me to develop a set of working ethical principles. There will be a need to keep these principles rather vague and general as they are expressions not of clear thought alone but of highly motivated pursuit of perfection. This pursuit of perfection itself, as in Smith, is a guarantee that we are basically ethically correct.

In Reid this pursuit of perfection is basically a felt and exercised drive to make the irrational rational. In this he is again different from Smith in wanting to grant a more major place to intellectual reasoning even though this reasoning is so strongly guided by a strong will. So while Smith would want us to focus on the emotional dimensions of a particular problematic case, Reid wants us to make as much rational sense out of it as we can. Our basic underlying general principles of ethics will help us to perceive the intellectual structures of the present case. Only when we have as completely as possible understood the complexities of the case as well as empathized with them have we fully and properly practiced ethics.

Sue is a 20-year-old woman who has been retarded since birth. She was born seven weeks prematurely, the first child of an unwed, 19-year-old mother. Because of Sue's prematurity a public health nurse was sent to the home to be sure adequate facilities and care were available for her. These things were found to be adequate. The family, however, was described as "disinterested." Sue's mother immediately turned Sue over to Sue's 72-year-old great-grandmother who totally cared for Sue until April, 1985 when Sue was returned to her mother. By now great-grandmother is 92 years old and no longer able to care for Sue.

Sue is friendly and outgoing and has become hyperactive. She frequently wanders away from home and has been returned by friends and even strangers. She does not take, or is not given, her phenobarbital for her seizures appropriately. Her phenobarbital levels are frequently subtherapeutic and sometimes too high. At least once she was treated for a massive overdose. Sue now attends a day care center for the retarded. She is cared for by her 16-year-old normal sister, while her mother works as a nurses' aid.

Review of Sue's chart reveals sporadic medical care with about 75 per cent of doctor's appointments not kept. There are numerous ER visits for minor problems and one bout with broncho-pneumonia. Chromosomal studies revealed no abnormalities. Intelligence testing at age six years placed her IQ at less than 50 on the WISC in all areas and overall. Sue is able to dress and feed herself but otherwise functions at the level of a two-year-old child.

Her problems are vaginal itching, metromenorrhagia, cyclic breast pain and anemia. Sue experienced menarche at age ten and always had heavy, irregular periods making hygiene difficult. She had been found running down the street or playing with blood on her clothes and legs. Her mother was quite concerned about this problem, but seemed much more concerned about the possibility that Sue might become pregnant. She stated that Sue had poor judgment and might be "taken advantage of." She knew Sue couldn't care for an infant and that she herself could not because she had to work to support Sue, her 16-year-old and herself. She inquired about the possibility of performing a hysterectomy on Sue to eliminate the poor hygiene, the anemia and the possibility of pregnancy.

Review of systems were negative. There was no history of gastrointestinal blood loss. Physical examination of Sue was normal. She appeared well-nourished (168lbs), but her mother states Sue won't eat meat. Pelvic exam was normal, but not an optimal exam because of Sue's lack of cooperation. Stool guaiac was negative. Laboratory studies were normal except for classic iron deficiency anemia. Serum 12 and whole blood folate levels were normal.

Clearly this is a complex situation. It calls for a great deal of sympathy and empathy on the part of health care professionals. But it also calls for a clear-headed use of moral principles to provide a structure for the information and allow some amount of simplicity. What values do you think this case elicits?

Rather like Smith's self-command the exercise of will is very crucial in Reid. Also, as in Smith, this exercise of will is central to the practice of virtue. Reid presents our thinking processes as being much controlled by habitual activities. We think in certain habitual patterns because we have beliefs which move us into these patterns. Our beliefs are the results of our decisions and commitments. But the prime role of will in the development of intellectual habits of thought is to make sure that irrational instincts are controlled and put at the service of mind.[29] Since the will is an active power cognate to instinctual drives, it can bend those drives into other more intellectual channels.

In this day of such specialization in medicine the decision to work in one area rather than another necessarily means that a physician will know less about other fields. As one goes along in the practice of medicine over many years lack of knowledge of parallel developments in other specialties can be a very serious problem. There is an instinctual move to diagnose and prognose along familiar lines. It is easy to miss or mistake patient symptoms. There has to be a decision to move outside the specialty and seek consult from another quarter. The same dynamics often work in the seeking or non-seeking of an ethical consult. At times the instinctive commitment to one or another course of treatment may blind us to other questions involved. If we really want to know more, we have to want to know more and decide to take action. Often our instincts push us to remain more complacent.

A practice of the virtue of benevolence would push us to go regularly and habitually the extra mile so as to best serve the patient. In the ranking of benevolence above justice in the catalog of virtues Reid agrees again with Hutcheson and Smith.[30] More strongly than both of them, however, Reid stresses that the role and function of will decision is to make the intellectual factors strong and operative. An example of this would be the situation where all or a number of the precise reasons why a course of action is being pursued are for the moment lost or obscure. We would continue on a particular course of action none the less because there is a firm decision that this course, for reasons which were better or more clearly known in the past, is the correct course.[31]

We have a set of benevolent instinctual emotions with which the will can cooperate in aiding our habitually rational approach. Some of these are pity and compassion, esteem of wisdom and goodness, friendship.[32] While this list is clearly incomplete Reid uses it to give examples of the kind of experiences which we have that we can build upon to perfect our ethical behavior. These emotions and the decisions to use them are also allied to an innate sense of duty or conscience.[33] The workings of these instinctual elements of will, emotion and conscience guide and direct the workings of practical reason.[34] This is the kind of skilled knowledge regularly used in both medicine and ethics. But Reid is concerned that even at its best this kind of knowledge can make numerous mistakes. So he says that there is another kind of knowledge, speculative knowledge. We should always be aiming at this kind of more precise and abstract knowledge.[35] Such knowledge would get at the more ultimate principles of medical or ethical knowledge. Since Reid's version of Newtonianism led him to believe (in his own specialized sense of belief) that these principles are really embedded in physical and mental reality, our knowledge of them would be of the truth itself. While we will not want to go that far in practice we rightly do hold up rather lofty intellectual ideals for our pursuit. This is vital lest the everyday practice of medicine and ethics narrows our view too much. There must be something always in principle above and beyond what we now know.

In the ethical sphere an emphasis on the speculative aspect of the ethical enterprise would lead us to classify the virtues along the familiar lines of prudence, justice, fortitude and temperance.[36] But Reid wants to keep this kind of ethics more idealistic and rather have us concentrate on ethics as we really experience it. Here our experience of virtuous actions would include feelings of honesty, disinterestedness, honor, rectitude.[37] The list is in no way meant to be exhaustive, but rather to give some sense of what it feels like to practice virtue not just to speculate about it.

Reid works very hard to strike a balance between instinctual emotive experiences and intellectual endeavor. He has a strong inclination to stress the former because he has a picture of the human being as being very actively involved in the affairs of work and life. Such a person is strong willed and driven to seek ever greater perfection. It is this exercise of inner drives which Reid thinks is the root and source of ethics. He even goes so far as to say that actions are moral, immoral or indifferent when we believe them to be so.[38] By this he does not mean at all to make ethics a matter of subjective capriciousness but rather to stress the dynamic quality of human striving and commitment. Our basic beliefs drive us toward ever better ethical behavior. This approach to ethics is particularly useful in dealing with professions such as medicine which so obviously are a kind of calling and vocation with many of the features of belief as Reid describes them.

But, while Reid wants to emphasize most the experience and exercise of these beliefs and decisions, he thinks that they operate in a wider context which is in fact the highly ordered Newtonian world of which we are all a part. The wider context assures objectivity, but we seldom have direct access to this context. Rather we can and should look more closely at the daily practical experience of practice to get in touch with our beliefs and motives so that we can better and constantly develop and perfect that practice. It is a strongly pragmatic approach which will be forged into a very powerful and effective moral tool by William James and John Dewey.

5

AMERICAN PRAGMATISM

The precise influence of Scottish Enlightenment philosophy on American thought is difficult to trace. But the use of a large number of manuals of philosophy in the Scottish style made it a rather constant presence. Certain of its themes were commonplace. Undoubtedly one of the major reasons for this was its basic compatibility with the American experience. There was a need to be simple, follow common sense, develop a clear and straight-forward ethics. The basic practicality of the Scots was most congenial to the American practice of fundamental know-how. A pragmatic philosophy would be the best. While this approach was used by a number of American thinkers two of the most important of them in terms of ethics are James and Dewey.

William James is far too unique and creative a genius to situate him too precisely in any tradition, but there are some strains of the pragmatist program that can be noted in a special way in the development of his thought. James was a moody and often depressed individual. He struggled much against this so that there is in his published writings a verve and optimism which would belie the circumstances of his personal life. One of his strongest remedies against himself was a strong belief in his own creative worth and power. James also exercised this belief in a strongly Reidian way in that he needed at key times of strife to make a strong and clear decision to have this belief.[1] It was a decision not based on any good reasons, indeed it in a certain way had to fly in the face of reason. So if we ask ourselves why we should be moral, the answer would be that our firm resolve to assert our belief and faith in ourselves is the only basically possible way to deal with this question.

But just as Reid had his grand scheme of the master mechanical

Newtonian as the ultimate guarantee of personalist ethics, so James believes not only in himself but in a sort of mystical all-embracing reality to which each of our staunch resolve contributes.[2] This is much bound up with a basic religious view in which James sees God as a transcendent being who is basically hidden from us. We can only get some knowledge and experience of divinity by being involved in some sort of mystical apprehension and activity. How seriously James took this is evidenced by what many consider to be his finest work, *The Varieties of Religious Experience*.

While this religious background is critical in understanding James, the pragmatism for which he is so famous demands that we not try to understand the divine reasons for things but rather that we simply believe that our best efforts are part of a large master plan. If we knew that plan we would not be in the situation of having to make such strong resolves. Any meanings which we grasp cannot come from the elusive divine planner but must be created by our own selves with the blind faith that they are part of that plan. Practically and pragmatically this means that in terms of our own experience we create our own meanings. This makes it necessary for resolve not only to triumph over intellect but in a certain sense to create knowledge itself.

There are privileged moments of resolve. These are times of unprecedented cases and lonely emergencies. Often in these cases we make unusual and unprecedented decisions which we cannot justify with anything like complete rationality.[3]

Medicine is a highly developed art and skill. There is no absolute body of knowledge to which we can go to solve difficult cases. Our textbooks are not directly authored by God. We are regularly confronted by unprecedented cases and lonely emergencies. (As I was actually typing up this paragraph my phone rang and I was called in as an ethical consultant on a problematic obstetrics case. I'm feeling just a little lonely and scared at this time. William James, I hear you.) In these situations we often go on our best instinct and hunch. It takes a great deal of courage and resolve to do this. We are often extremely fearful of the conseqeuences of what we have to do. But we are not God, so we have to make the most meaningful decision we can in the case in the hope that it fits into some larger medical, moral and divine plan.

James also notes that these decisions can often be some of the very best that we make. The resolve to try to do our best can open up some possibilities which we had not previously considered. The history of medicine is filled with dramatic breakthroughs which have occurred only in crisis situations. What never occurred to us to try or what seemed in other circumstances to be too dangerous and untried turns out to be the best procedure for cure or care. Moral miracles also occur in these circumstances. New and fresh resolutions of dilemmas are forged in the fire of frustration. James is quite explicit in noting that sickrooms may be the places for these privileged moments of moral revelation.[4]

In this kind of situation there is regularly a confusion brought about because of a conflict of principles. Rules of morality which seemed to have worked quite well in other contexts fail us now. No single one of them yields an answer. What is needed is a fusion or combination of principles. James refers to it as a chemical combination among these principles.[5] Parts of principles have to meld and blend in new ways so as to produce a way of action. We should not be dismayed that we must give way on old principles but rather see that these principles have not died but are conceived, gestated and then reborn into new moral life. A growing ease with the multiplicities of life will take us ever into more moral richness.

There are often several technically "correct" approaches to treatment. The decision to opt for one approach rather than another sometimes flows from the sympathy physicians have for their patients. Consider the following situation.

Mr. D., an 86-year-old man who has been bedridden for two years in a nursing home after a stroke, is now suffering from very painful decubitus ulcers on his back and buttocks, weighs less than 85lbs, and is severely aphasic and paralyzed on the right side. He has developed a fever that spiked to 105°F, is severely congested, and his attending physician, Dr. Kay, has diagnosed pneumonia. Mr. D. had had pneumonia once before since the stroke, but had recovered after aggressive treatment. It is now 4.30 a.m. and Dr. Kay orders a urine culture and chest X-ray to confirm his diagnosis.

Mr. D. has no living relatives or friends, except Dr. Kay, who has been his physician since the original stroke. Dr. Kay knows that his patient has expressed to him and to nursing home personnel the wish not to be kept alive by any means possible if recovery is remote. But he wished to die with dignity when the time comes. But he's now not competent to make decisions for himself and, although he had previously requested that a Do Not Resuscitate order be placed in his record, Dr. Kay is not now faced with that decision. Rather he must decide whether or not he should treat Mr. D.'s present crisis aggressively.

He reflects on his own beliefs and feelings. He believes that if he were Mr. D. he would not want aggressive treatment. But he also believes he would not want to suffer. Furthermore, as a physician, Dr. Kay is professionally committed to doing something, but he is not committed to doing everything possible.

He decides not to transfer Mr. D. to the hospital where he would be treated in a "technically correct" way. Nor does he administer penicillin or tell the nursing home to encourage fluid uptake. Instead, letting his sympathy for Mr. D.'s plight and his beliefs about the patient's expressed wishes aid him in making a decision, Dr. Kay tells the staff only to keep him as comfortable as possible and to do nothing else.

All three alternatives may be technically correct, but only in the last case does one's sympathy take main control. This isn't to say the decision is irrational. Sympathy can, however, interact with what we know and justifiably believe about patients' wishes. To withhold sympathy can be a way of refusing to treat patients as persons rather than as objects to be manipulated.

Because of the searing and dramatic aspect of these decisions they tend to strongly personally affect us. They tend to contribute sharply to the development of our character. James has a good deal to say about character. This is his version in a way of virtue ethics. Our character will determine how we will ethically respond. It plays a vital role in a crisis situation. But character is never to be habitual in the sense of being dull and routine. Rather we must be constantly choosing just what kind of character we want to have.[6]

There is a very strong social dimension to James' ethical thought. He was a crusader for all sorts of social goods such as the rights of women, blacks and other minorities. He was against unrestricted capitalism. He was in favor of allowing the practice of non-traditional medicine. All of this was intimately connected with his version of moral sympathy. Unlike the Hume version which was rather a mechanical view of human interaction based in large part on the sheer fact of personal proximity, James' sympathy was grounded in the vital need to overcome a degree of pessimism which could lead to suicidal tendencies. Against this pessimism James noted that the exercise of my determined will to survive and excel is done in the context of my noting that I am a part of the brotherhood of humanity. We recognize that we are all involved in a struggle to do the best with this very difficult human situation in which we find ourselves. This makes us feel a profound sympathy with each other. It also makes us experience a deep drive to do the best we can to help each other out.[7]

While this sounds more than a bit dramatic, it often really is the situation in the practice of medicine. Hospitals are places of constant heroism on the part of patients and medical staff. There is such a sense of sympathy that one has to take measures not to get too caught up in the emotion of it. There is also all around you the temptation to give up in the face of terrible odds. We are constantly motivated to do our best in trying to help in what we know are impossible situations. The struggle is regularly titanic. This exercise of heroic sympathy adds the specifically ethical element to the medical situation. Without it we may be practicing medicine only or primarily as the exercise of technical skill. The physician who is only or primarily just a technician may have found this way of operating so as to be insulated from the trauma of involvement but the level of medicine practiced in this way will be considerably lower than medicine practiced with sympathetic concern. This is so because the medical situation actually and really is not one of sheer or basic technology but rather one of important if intense human interaction. Treating it as primarily technology is untrue to the realities of the medical encounter. Even the rather remote radiologist or pathologist is dealing with the severe life and death struggles of the patients. Attention to and cultivation of sympathy will insure that a strong and vibrant ethical force runs through medical practice and makes it the involved and caring profession all civilizations and cultures hold it to be. Radiologists often have to deal, usually reluctantly, with the following type of problem.

Mrs. James went to her family physician because she had noticed a lump in her left breast. He examined her and told her that the lump might be malignant but that she needed to take some further diagnostic tests including X-rays. She had the tests performed and then was told to return for the results in three days.

During that time she had worked herself into a frenzy. She was terrified that the tests might be positive so she went to the hospital the next day to see if she could find out anything. Her physician was not there so she went to see the radiologist.

It turned out to be a very difficult confrontation for both of them because the radiologist did in fact have the results of her X-rays. They were positive. In this case the radiologist believed that

Mrs. James was in very bad psychological shape and needed to know what he could tell her. He did not want her to have to wait until the next day because he felt suddenly very sympathetic to her plight. He encouraged her to talk to her own physician as soon as possible but explained the results of the test and provided her with some initial information on treatment modes and their success rates.

While one of the appeals of radiology is the absence of such encounters, patients nonetheless have a right to the truth and it is often kinder to provide the truth as soon as possible than to wait until a more "appropriate" physician can do so.

Along with this concern for sympathy there is in James a stress on optimism. He is convinced that the rigid adherence to principles is the source of pessimism. Our principles just do not neatly fit every situation. They especially do not fit critical and problematic situations. The very fact that they do not fit is, of course, precisely what makes these situations problematic. We can say that in these circumstances the principles still hold but there are exceptions. But this will not get us out of the basic gloom of not being able really to understand or cope with the data.[8] Rather we have to be ready and anxious to note that there really are different things which we confront.

James expressed this rather constant appearance of new and challenging situations in evolutionary terms. He was deadly against any deterministic interpretation of Darwin. Rather the experience of evolution shows that there are always unpredictable spontaneous variations. It is the breaking out of old ways which is the vitality and life of evolution. Movement forward is its essence. But we have to be always careful not to pretend to know the whole plan and picture. To know this would rob us of the experience of spontaneity as we would already know the answers. Rather the most exhilarating and exciting experience for us is to participate in the creative energy of variation and change. All of these changes have an ethical dimension. The highly principled ethician is gloomy about change, defensive of staunch positions, suspicious of progress, vicious in attacking enemies. The pragmatic ethical optimist delights in the freshness of change, new advances and creative approaches, embraces progress and is ever alert to acquire new friends. The fact that we find the world imperfect is not a cause for grief and gloom. Rather than lamenting that imperfection will not go away, the acceptance of it gives us something to do. We are to battle to improve an imperfect world.

If a physician is going to be happy in medical practice, then it is necessary to adopt Jamesian optimism. We are constantly confronted by often some of the most glaring imperfections of the human condition. Most people try to deny or at least avoid these situations. The physician makes them an integral part of life. The struggle to overcome medical problems makes physicians among the most moral and ethical of humans. But, fine psychologist which he was, James also notes that we cannot so throw ourselves into this endeavor as to have no time for calm and repose. At these moments we also recognize our limitations. One of the functions of philosophy is to provide these moments of repose and reflection.

The philosopher is often presented in caricature as the person of infinite repose. We sit in our ivory towers and quietly contemplate the world. Some are so convinced that this caricature is in fact the reality that they cannot imagine how a philosopher can possibly be involved in such a complex and puzzling activity as the practice of medicine.

James' position is that everyone, philosopher or physician, must be reflective and active. But medicine pulls the physician towards ever more activity so that reflection is a problem. Philosophy lures one to somnolent contemplation. While it is very difficult to strike the balance individually, a team effort might have a better chance. The rounding clinical medical ethicist can provide a measure of reflective assessment of the situation denied to the harried practitioner. But the ethicist must be drawn as deeply as possible into the responsibilities of medical practice so as to be able to make sure that whatever principles or approaches are being taken are not remote and aloof but clear, precise and effective.

Mr. B. is a patient at Lakeside Veterans Administration Center. He is 54 years old. He has a history of alcohol abuse, no family and no job. He was admitted to the VA with ulcerative colitus which has been treated sufficiently for him to be released but he had suffered a heart attack the previous week.

During walk-around rounds Dr. Jones, the VA's new ethicist, looked at Mr. B.'s chart and did not see an order for a social work consult. The VA, Dr. Jones knew, has a rule that states that a hospital social worker has to interview each patient within two days of admission. Nonetheless it looked to Dr. Jones as if very little had been done to facilitate Mr. B.'s discharge planning. This was an oversight probably caused by the enormous patient load at Lakeside, but it was an important one for a patient like Mr. B. who would require nursing home care for several weeks and had not personal resources to finance such expensive extended care.

Dr. Jones exercised his authority to write a note in the patient's chart ordering a social work consult and in the progress notes he emphasized the need to begin discharge planning for Mr. B. as soon as possible.

While James certainly wants to stress optimism as the best approach in ethics, he does not want us to be naive about this. So he sometimes speaks of meliorism as midway between optimism and pessimism.[9] This is not meant to be a pernicious mean between these two extremes but rather to point out the need for constant striving to attain the best possible result. If we hold out optimism simply as an ideal we might fall into the trap of thinking that we know too well just what this optimum might be. We would grow complacent in having attained our goal when much remains to be done. Meliorism keeps us carefully and precisely working within the pragmatic parameter of what can be attained.

But James' melioristic optimism contains a very strong degree of striving for perfection. He makes this a very strong inner feeling. If we have a sense that we are doing the best that we can, then the chances are that we are acting ethically. This sense he compares to the sense of taste. The better thing tastes better.[10] Deeply felt desires such as these intensify into moral imperatives.[11]

This factor of perfectionism makes James' ethic particularly applicable to medical practice. Given the immense progress still to be made in medicine and the dire need to be able to do the best we can in curing patients now in critical need, we have to keep constantly striving for the best we can do under the circumstances. Perfectionism is built right into medical practice.

What is true of perfectionism in medical practice is also true of perfectionism in the practice of medical ethics. The medical ethician who thinks that an ultimate solution has been reached in a particular case or set of cases must be overlooking a number of factors which should be a spur to ever better ethics. Purely and simply, ethical complacency is bad ethics. It leaves a bad taste in the mouth. The pursuit of perfection rather demands a thirst for ever better ethics.

Dr. Jones, the consultant in medical ethics at Memorial Hospital, has been asked to join a discussion of a very troubling situation. A 36-year-old man with HIV infection had been admitted a week earlier becuse he had attempted to commit suicide by swallowing a toxic dose of a narcotic drug. Henry did not yet have full-blown AIDS but, according to his roommate and lover, had become very depressed when he contemplated the likelihood that he would eventually develop AIDS. Henry was now so mentally and physically disabled that he could not move or speak although his EEG registered cortical activity.

Henry has been a very independent, creative man who made a living as an artist. Tom, the roommate, has been his constant companion for three years and has won in court the right to act as Henry's surrogate. Tom has insisted that Henry would not want to continue living with so little of his cognitive and physical capabilities and that he had tried to commit suicide even before the most recent attempt. Tom wants Henry's life support systems and all other medical treatment to be terminated including antibiotics and nutrition.

Henry's prognosis is unclear. Nobody can say for sure whether or not he has reached a plateau. The nurses working with Henry believe he has started to communicate a little non-verbally in the last few days and have argued that medical treatment should continue at least for a little while longer. The resident has seen no improvement and considers Tom's legal and moral authority to be incontrovertible. Dr. Barnowski, Henry's attending physician, is unwilling to make definite predictions about Henry's future although he is inclined to agree with the nurses. At the conference the following dialog ensued.

Dr. B.: If treatment is terminated Henry will certainly not improve and will probably die within a week. He doesn't have AIDS yet and I wonder if we can be certain he has reached a plateau.

R.: But the roommate wants treatment to be stopped and we don't have good reasons to believe he does not know Henry's interests or have them as his primary concern. Tom is making the decisions for Henry and it is only through him that we can tell what Henry's own preferences would be if he could express them. Patient autonomy is the ideal we should be striving for and this is the closest we can get. And it seems pretty clear that Henry did not want to live with the prospect of AIDS anyway.

N.: If Henry is even slightly improved we should give him a chance to get well enough to make his own decisions.

Dr. J.: I agree with R. that autonomy should not be violated but it seems to me that we should not jump to the conclusion that autonomy would best be served by stopping all medical treatment at this point. We may want to ensure that Henry's life be extended a while longer to make sure he has reached a plateau. Also we might find out we don't know everything there is to know about Henry's preferences. I suggest we provide minimal support such as nutrition and antibiotics, but that we do not interfere if there is a crisis.

Reluctantly the resident agreed and they persuaded Tom to allow them to pursue that course. Henry's condition improved slightly in the weeks that followed and eventually he was able to communicate enough to let the medical team know he wanted to go home.

One very interesting feature of this situation is that Henry's wish to die, which had figured in the resident's argument, turned out to be less certain than Tom had believed. During the discussions with Tom following the first conference he admitted that Henry had called him at work the day he swallowed the pills to find out if and when Tom would be home. As it happened Tom was delayed and arrived home two hours later than he had anticipated. That information was relevant to the heretofore unquestioned assumption that Henry really wanted to die.

Dr. Jones' suggestion that they may be violating Henry's autonomy by assuming too quickly that they knew how to maximize it had the result that further discussion revealed more about Henry's wishes than Tom was able initially to provide.

The moral sense kind of theme noted in James' perfectionism motif also plays a strong part in the relation James sees between ethics and aesthetics. This connection has roots in the Scottish tradition. Hutcheson, for instance, along with his development of the theory of moral sense was much interested in the question of the development of an aesthetic sense. There are two key reasons why James linked the aesthetic and ethical sense. First of all he pointed out that aesthetic principles play a cognitive role in any intellectual endeavor.[12] A good investigation or proof has a certain elegance about it, a certain cleanness.

The solution of complex diagnostic or prognostic problems often has this character to it. Why go along one diagnostic route rather than another? There is a certain elegance to it. It has a certain rhythm or pattern. It looks better. The successful conclusion of the surgical or medical procedure is often greeted with cries of

"Beautiful, beautiful." Not just idle chatter but a strongly felt emotive exclamation of the aesthetic.

The second reason James had for blending the aesthetic and ethic was the matter of style. A task carried out with a certain flair or style would be an indication that the proper skill was being competently exercised. The whole medical team is uncomfortable in the presence of a timid and hesitant physician. They should be equally ill at ease with a timid ethicist. Since so much of the practice of ethics and medicine is a skill, art here is not a luxury but integrally part of the process.

But there are two considerations which give ethics a priority over aesthetics. First, aesthetics is much more inchoate and intuitive than ethics. It is very difficult to develop rules for art. But, even though there is the strong creative thrust in ethics, it does work with principles, rules and argumentation. Here again ethics is more like medicine. The brilliant intuitive diagnostician must provide reasons for the course of action. Those reasons must somehow come out of or at least relate to the traditional practice of medicine in the case. Ethical traditions must also work into any new creative approach. As much as possible clear argumentation must bolster insight.

Secondly, ethical activity culminates in a choice of greater consequence than an aesthetic option. This is so because ethical choice is so obviously committed to the attempt to cure the deficiencies of an imperfect world. Aesthetics sets out not so much to cure as to delight. Aesthetics can start from what is good and make it better. Ethics usually comes upon a bad situation and tries to improve it. But it is important to not see ethics as just solving a problem. This would make it too minimalistic. All it would do is resolve a bad situation as best as possible, but still leave the situation bad. It would just say what is permissible to be done in dire circumstances. Rather more positively an ethical solution should bring good out of a bad situation, hold out hope for the future, bring beauty out of ugliness. An ethical solution which does nothing but basically untangle problems is only at best half true, at worst quite false. Ethics must always hold out the beauty of hope.

Liver cancer has until recently been considered virtually impossible to check. In relatively advanced stages it is resistant to chemotherapy and has been considered almost inoperative. Hence the prognosis for someone with liver cancer has been poor.

101

But the situation is changing especially with respect to surgical techniques. Skilled surgeons can now remove several points on the liver at which cancer is located without causing liver failure.

When Joe, a 54-year-old steelworker, checked into Memorial Hospital suffering from liver cancer he had become very depressed. He considered cancer to be virtually a death sentence and his family doctor had told him that liver cancer had a poor prognosis. He came to Memorial for a work-up and the attending told him a different story.

"First of all, Joe, many cancers, including lung cancer, can now be treated even in middle stages with some degree of success. Chemotherapy can at least prolong life with relatively high quality for several years longer than was the case 15 years ago.

But even though liver cancer doesn't respond well to chemotherapy a skilled surgeon can remove several areas on the liver and the liver will still function well. I don't want to give you any false hope because the surgical techniques are so new there is not a large data base for making prognoses, but I can tell you about several recent liver cancer patients in this area who have recovered sufficiently after surgery performed during the past year to go home and live relatively normal lives.

So I'm going to suggest some things you can do to help yourself. First, tell your family what I've just told you. I'll give you some literature on the subject to take to them. You'll need their support. Second, we'll administer chemotherapy until the operation if you choose to go that route. But at the same time I want you to make a list of all the things you get the most pleasure doing. And each day I want you to do at least one of the things on that list."

Sometimes being ill can move us to appreciate those aspects of our lives that we most cherish. At the same time such an appreciation can help us to recover from our illness. This is something Joe's hospital physician knows.

The theme of hope is strong in James. It is much connected to his fascination with things religious. So strong is our felt need to commit ourselves to the perfection of our human possibilities that we have to see ourselves in cooperation with a power of ultimate creative hope. There is a real sense of some sort of transcendent reality which we can never see clearly at any time, but which must be there in order for us to find meaning at all for the pedestrian pragmatic tasks which we encounter every day.[13]

The root of Jamesian religiosity is in the strong personal commitment we make to improve and live our life to the best and fullest degree of which we are capable. This places him securely in the tradition of mystical religion. The mystic is through and through a person with a strong sense of prayer. But the prayer is not primarily for the aesthetic delight of it. While aesthetics is certainly there, the main purpose of prayer is the bringing about of personal conversion. This conversion involves the taking of certain very concrete actions to bring about good in the world. The mystic who so withdraws from the world as to make no real contribution to it is suspect indeed. Rather those most often admired in various religious traditions are the people who strike a balance between prayer and action rather like the balance noted before between ethical reflection and activity.

But the mystic quality of religious experience also serves as a brake on the too literal application of religious materials to the solution of ethical problems. Since religious expectations are so much framed in highly imaginative aesthetic language and art they have the power to give us strong motivation to action. But a too literal application of religious statements and experience from other times and other cultures can usurp the legitimate functions of ethics which tries to grapple as best as possible with problems here and now. Importation of too many religious principles and their transformation into ethical principles can lead to a pessimistic ethics of principles.

A great strength of mystical religion is that it strikes such a strongly felt personal chord. Essential to any ethics is this inner drive to excellence. It is rare and difficult to sustain this drive over long periods of time in the absence of any type of religiosity at all.

In the times of crisis and strife so often confronted in the practice of medicine, physician, patient and family find themselves reaching for religious dimensions. The ethicist, too, needs to have this felt drive to be in touch with what is best in reality. Religion at its best is an experience of undeterred and ultimate hope. The greatest privilege possible given to the clinical ethicist is to be able to participate in the physician's power to bring the possibilities of hope in even the most problematic of medical crises. If this hope is not provided then the practice of ethical pragmatism is hollow and empty. We come into people's lives at a time when we have the chance to move them and ourselves to a higher plane of activity and awareness. The best of us is what they always deserve.

Dr. Jones, the ethics consultant at Memorial Hospital, has worked very hard for five years. He is often on 24-hour call. He has worked very hard to keep abreast of both philosophical and clinical literature and writes several major papers a year. In addition he donates some of his time and energy to a local AIDS support group and lectures community organizations on aspects of clinical ethics. In short, he is exhausted.

Dr. Jones has lately started to drink a little too much. He justifies this behavior by telling himself that he needs some way to wind down each day as quickly as possible so he can get enough sleep. But his colleagues have noticed a change in the way in which he interacts with them during rounds and conferences. He seems to "space out" as one resident put it to her supervising physician and everyone noticed that he was starting to clutch when there was pressure on him to provide a reasoned solution to a tough ethical problem.

Several of his colleagues have met to discuss how to approach Dr. Jones with their concern about what they have come to believe is a drinking problem. Some didn't want to approach him at all, but others were concerned both about his health and the well-being of their patients.

This is not a situation that is easy to deal with in a hospital. An ego is easily bruised and when health care professionals are in trouble they tend to cover it up. But in this case, Dr. Jones himself had become aware of his problems. He knew that he owed responsibilities first to patients and then to colleagues. He knew that he was abrogating those responsibilities, but most important, as he came to realize one night while reflecting on the difficulties he'd had concentrating that day, he had responsibilities to himself. Being as fully involved in the clinical process as possible is an important part of making his life go well. The next day, Dr. Jones made an appointment with a psychiatrist on staff. He needed to regain his sense of vitality and optimism.

Pragmatism is suffused with a sense of buoyant optimism. This is clearly seen in the massive work of the quintessential American pragmatist, John Dewey. There is the hope that just about any problem can be solved if only we can get a basic methodology to come to grips with it and then have the desire and tenacity to continue to work. So through the long course of his career Dewey took on the task of solving questions not only in philosophy but also in psychology, education and society.

Like William James his starting point, however, is psychology. So there is an early outline or syllabus of ethics called *The Study of Ethics: A Syllabus*. After a rather short introduction on the nature of ethical theory which breaks it down into practical encouragement and discouragement of certain acts, urging restraint through speech and reflective judgment, the vast majority of the text is taken up with the study of the psychological bases of ethics.[14] This begins by saying that all conduct is at first impulsive.[15] But we must learn to understand and control this kind of impulsive behavior. Like James, Dewey sought to find a linkage between conceptual psychological experience and the new findings about the material structure of the brain and nervous system. He was much taken with the patterns of the reflex arc as noted in the operations of sensation. This involves a stimulus, a central process of awareness and a motor response.[16] This tripartite approach will run through practically all of Dewey's thought. We first must confront a problem. This provides a stimulus for our actions. There follows a grappling with the complexities of the situation and then an intelligently responsive solution.

This pattern is central to both of the major ethics texts which, in collaboration with James Tufts, Dewey produced in 1908 and 1932.[17] These texts contain a good deal of historical material which is primarily by Tufts and carefully worked out methodology sections which are by Dewey.

The role of ethics as impulse is very strong in the 1908 *Ethics*. Reality itself is here perceived as a kind of a living dynamic unity with a set of inner drives. There is a tendency in reality to a kind of self-perfection. As a result our basic felt ethical impulses are experienced to be a movement toward always the better. The good is held out as a shining ideal toward which we tend. But this tendency is not without its problems so we must constantly strive to improve ourselves. Rights and duties come into ethics as mechanisms reminding us of directions to be taken and paths to be followed. They are more directly concerned with the building up of a personal ethics.[18] Virtues are traits of character which support the common good.[19] But the emphasis in this text remains more on the satisfaction of self in productive enterprise.

Medical practice is a very idealistic sort of endeavor. We often picture it as achieving ever more and more good. Indeed we do not often question at all if the advance of medicine itself is an unmitigated good. We take that for granted. Any progress we make in medicine must automatically be for the good. The rights of patients and the duties of physicians are seen in the light of the larger good of the whole enterprise. Habitual patterns of action on the part of physicians at least are taken to be useful in serving the common good of both physicians and patients. Some caution must be observed in this kind of projected view of medicine in that we might not be so concerned to question in detail a number of the precise rights, duties or virtues. This will tend to make our ethics quite vague and based on wider unexamined presuppositions. There is also the possibility of a good deal of selfishness being involved in that we follow too uncritically our inner impulsive drives and presume that they are leading us to the good. Social aspects of the practice of medicine tend to be made subservient to personal professional goals. The physician's drive to succeed and excel may turn out to be more central to medical and ethical practice than the needs and goods of the patient.

The 1932 *Ethics* presents a much more pragmatic interaction between individual and society.[20] One is seen as the function of the other. The role of habits and virtues is strengthened in this configuration. More precise attention is paid to the practical details of personal and professional interaction. The change in emphasis is anchored, however, in the tripartite structure first noted in the workings of the reflex arc. The psychological emphasis of that work led to a viewing of the 1908 ethical project as being grounded in self-enhancing impulses, a development of social virtues or habits, and an intelligent resolution of practical questions. The 1932 ethical project starts rather with the situation of human needs, works through the type of customs which have developed in dealing with these problems, and tries to reach a new and creative solution to the questions. This last move is the rather famous reconstructive turn in Dewey's philosophy.

Just as there are these two moves in Dewey's thought the same kind of dynamic may be seen operative in the development of American medicine. For most of its history the emphasis was on the development of personal medical and ethical skills on the part of the practitioner. An examination of the early codes of medical ethics would rather clearly show that social questions were secondary to problems of the internal development of the profession itself. When the resources and techniques of medicine were still rather limited it is understandable that this would be the case. But the situation now is much different. Medicine is a highly established social phenomenon in this country. It has its own needs which may not coincide precisely with the needs of patients. It has built up a considerable set of customs as to how to deal with a wide variety of cases. There are many calls from many quarters for rather radical reconstructions of many aspects of medical practice.

Consider the problem of Dr. Humphries and Judy Wiggins. Judy is a 45-year-old nurse at Memorial Hospital who had contracted cardiomyopathy. She had been given a very poor prognosis and she had written a living will instructing her caretakers to refrain from using extraordinary means to keep her alive. As it turned out, her left ventricle stopped functioning and Dr. Humphries, Memorial's chief surgeon, ordered her to be placed on a left ventricle assist device. Mrs. Wiggins was now in a coma.

Dr. Humphries had a great deal of prestige both in the hospital and in the community. He had developed a very strong ego and did not take advice very well. He had the reputation within the hospital of, as one nurse put it, "not letting any of his patients die on his machine." And now Mrs. Wiggins was one of those patients.

Despite her living will, the advice of her family, the floor nurses, the chief resident and the ethics consultant to remove her from the left ventricle assist device, Mrs. Wiggins was maintained on the device for two weeks until she finally died. Dr. Humphries is a very skilled surgeon but he has become incapable of listening to what his patients and his staff believe are mistakes of judgment. Mrs. Wiggins' family has sued Dr. Humphries and Memorial Hospital for negligence and infringement of Mrs. Wiggins' civil rights.

Clearly Dr. Humphries has to deal better with his patterns of impulsive behavior. The work of John Dewey's middle period illuminates many aspects of this kind of behavior and situates it in the broader context of human ethical activity.

In 1922 John Dewey published an important work in ethics called *Human Nature and Conduct*. It signals the shift in his thinking from the 1908 to the 1932 *Ethics*. Here there is a re-working of an earlier ethical triad. While the previous view was founded first in biological drives, then proceeded to a consideration of the social consequences of these drives and finally to individual reflection about the two previous factors, the new view treats the biological factors in terms of a study of impulses and impulsive behavior, then proceeds to a study of the habitual regulation of these kinds of impulses in terms of a final study of the workings of human intelligence. Evident here is a move away from a somewhat deterministic Darwinian type of view towards a much more psychologically oriented approach. While the new triad is basically impulse, habit, intelligence, the book begins with the study of habit. Here there is a considerable study of habits as central to social functioning, the relation of character and conduct to habit, the role of customs in the shaping of morality. Rather than consider habitual action to be something which we individually develop in isolation from other people, Dewey is now strongly concerned to point out that really only in interaction with other people do our patterns of character and habit mature.

This view of habitual action is clearly seen and is indeed encouraged by the way in which young physicians are trained. Young people enter medical school with an almost biologically felt impulse to become physicians. Up to that point in their pre-medical training some of them under the pressure of attaining the good grades needed to allow them to enter medical school have even become loners. But the first few years of medical school force them into patterns of habitual activity which are dictated and controlled by the challenges and pressures of teamwork. This is only increased in the third and fourth year clerkships.

I teach (as part of a team) a first year medical ethics class. Two groups of students are required in a given week to thoroughly discuss two separate highly problematical medical ethical cases. They must assign different aspects of the case among themselves for study and research. The next week they must present the results of the study and the resolution of the case to the other group for criticism and comment. Hopefully this kind of activity will not only bring about the teamwork skills so necessary for medical practice but will also give individual students the opportunity to come to some self-realization as to what types of ethical choices they tend to make. Of most importance here would not so much be the actual decisions which are reached, but rather the perceived patterns of decision making. It would be important to know with as much clarity as possible what might be the underlying reasoning patterns involved in one's personal ethical decisions. It would be of considerable help if the individual decision maker could also situate these decisions in terms of some of the better known and developed theoretical approaches to ethics.

But Dewey is much concerned to point out that we seldom make practical decisions in terms of the rules of highly elaborate ethical systems. Rather we work our way much more intuitively through the details of particular cases, weighing and balancing many disparate factors until we come to some sort of a clarity. Rather than having a set of rigid ethical rules to which we adhere, we have rather a group of principles which are much more elusive and deeply ingrained in our individual character. We often speak of an individual as being a man or woman of principle, but we would be hard pressed to say just what precisely those principles are.

Doctors often rightly take pride in being people of principle. The many complex cases which they deal with so often on a regular basis over the course of many years of practice make them aware that they are deeply involved in ethics at almost all times. But there is a great deal of insecurity because of the inability to articulate with any degree of clarity the number and kind of principles on which they constantly and habitually operate.

In November of 1930 John Dewey read an address in English before the French Philosophical Society. It was first published in a French translation in 1930 and first published in an English translation from the French only in 1966.[21] This landmark article isolates three independent factors in morality. One is the notion of good; another is the role of laws; a third involves factors of praise or blame. Most important to note is that here Dewey may well be doing his most significant reconstructive move in ethics. This is because these factors are made to be completely independent. There is no attempt at all to correlate them and put them together. Practically speaking Dewey is trying to show that in our actual practice of ethical decision making we do not put various ethical elements together. Rather we have the personal experience of these factors as operating much more freely and independently. We do not experience ethical decision making as a clear and neatly coherent activity, rather we know that the process and the final decision leave many aspects of the matter unclear or not referred to at all. One or another aspect of the case pushes us one way or another in the decision.

Dewey does not want us to feel uneasy about the ambiguities of this, but rather to take it as the normal ethical situation. All ethics, but especially any practical applied ethics, cannot resolve all anomalies. The very nature of practicality means that ultimate abstract questions are not resolved. But this does not mean that practical ethical decisions are wrong or unfinished. It just means that they are practical.

Practical decisions in medical ethics are particularly experienced in this way. Almost all practical medical decisions, at least those in problematic cases, cannot appeal to neat and clear formulations of precise medical principles. Rather some medical aspects of the case remain problematic and unexplained. In critical care situations, some things may remain untreated as more pressing concerns demand action for acute problems. But some of the best medicine is often practiced precisely by focusing on the area of most critical need and allowing the other elements to remain in abeyance. By contrast an attempt to be too holistic and cure everything integrally at once would only lead to failure of the whole medical project.

The same would hold in ethical judgments. It is far better to be able to address the most pressing ethical problem and provide some solution rather than to try to handle all of the complexities of the case in a futile attempt to reach final and optimal ethical solutions. All of the rights and duties of all of the parties to a crucial ethical decision are seldom satisfied. But if the most important and central ones are met it is not only morally alright that others be ignored or played down, it is the only correct action we might take.

Critical in this new approach to ethics in Dewey is the fact that not only are moral conflicts not resolved but conflict itself becomes the very stuff of ethics. Ethical decisions are forged in the play of basically contrasting factors which cannot in principle be completely resolved. Any complete resolution of a case might signal that we have in fact reached a quite bad ethical conclusion. Dewey sees this conflict written large in the development historically of various types of opposing ethical theories. Ethical theories of a utilitarian type which emphasize the consequences of our actions in the pursuit of one or another type of ethical good are in conflict with deontological ethical theories which stress the prior role of principle and duty. Even within a particular ethical approach there are endless controversies as to which elements of the system should be given priority. Dewey thinks that there are strong social and political reasons why there is both a conflict between and within systems. Some social situations call more for the pursuit of goods or happiness, for instance, while others need to stress order, principle and duty. But we should not be surprised that we regularly appeal to seemingly contrasting ethical points of view. The situation might very well dictate just such an ethical eclecticism.

One of the services which our ethical team provides to the hospital and to the medical school is a regular set of ethical grand rounds. Here an actual case from medical practice is argued out before all interested physicians and students. Usually three points of view are presented. One may be by a physician, another by a lawyer and a third by an ethicist, or there may be two medical points of view and one ethical, or two ethical and one medical. Since these sessions are rigidly limited to one hour and as much time as possible is to be available for discussion, the initial presentations must be brisk and to the point. The presenters are required to come to some precise conclusions and make specific recommendations as to what should be done to resolve the case. There are usually sharp points of difference among the participants. While this format has worked well, a constant difficulty is that discussants are regularly accused of being dogmatically one-sided. Or they are accused of ethically pontificating as though they really know the only right answer and are set on imposing this solution on everyone. Often, if they have participated in other grand rounds presented to the same audience, their own self-contradicting arguments are brought bitingly to their attention.

It is extremely difficult to make clear that no participant in the discussion really does think that the answer to the medical or ethical dilemma is that clear. Rather in the interests of clarity and brevity a clear and concise stand is taken in order that further discussion and debate will be generated with the eventual hope that as many people as possible present will be able to formulate their own solution to the problem and give their own medical and ethical reasons for this solution. The point of the discussion is not so much to resolve the dilemma. By their very nature ethical dilemmas just do not admit of easy or of any solution. Rather the grand rounds is to juxtapose as many possible reasonable courses of action so that the dynamics of the debate are in themselves the solution.

While this may seem at first strange, a realization of the fiercely pragmatic nature of medicine will help to see that in actual practice this is what we really do in attacking and resolving medical ethical dilemmas. As a problematic case proceeds through diagnosis and prognosis many members of the health care team have an input. Seldom is this a situation where there is complete agreement as to aims and treatment. Especially if the case is a highly problematic one different opinions must be present and active. One or another intervention is pursued for a variety of reasons. The authority of the attending physician may be dominant. Patient or family wishes may override other considerations. Nursing staff may have severe reservations. The opinion of a consulting physician or ethicist or lawyer may be central. Social work might strongly impinge.

Conflicts are not so much resolved as certain steps taken in the very face of conflicting views. Social and political power bases usually determine when and how which moves will be made. But, as in the grand rounds situation, it is very important to be as aware as possible of the range of options and the grounds for those options. This assures that decisions made and actions taken will be in the context of as much knowledge and deliberation as possible. The very presence of this abundance of information is what makes the resolution of the medically moral problem ethical.

The serious entertaining of the conflicting possibilities is ethics. Not to pay any attention to these matters is unethical behavior. So we rightly chasten the imperious or impulsive individual who will not take into account other points of view. But, while we are required to take into account those points of view, it is impossible to act on all of them. In the course of a complicated case, we may try now one, now another tack. We often even do contradictory things. There is no one action we can take to solve a dilemma; rather we handle parts and pieces of it as best we can as the case unfolds.

We sometimes make the mistake of labeling a person unethical if an action is taken which is not in agreement with our perspective on the case. Really we might be much more unethical in such behavior in that we only see one aspect and expect this to be the ultimate solution. A person is unethical not because an action is taken contrary to a particular piece of advice, but because no effort is made to have as many as possible points of view present for consideration and selection. The more complex the case the more the need for more points of view. Conflict and controversy are the very stuff of ethics. A clear and easy resolution of a case may be the most unethical thing we can do. The stress on conflict and complexity which characterizes this mature phase of Dewey's ethical theory is also closely connected with the developing ethical role of virtue and character. Because character is so much a matter of type and temperament Dewey notes the strong role played by affective and emotive factors in personality development. But emotive factors tend to be much more inchoate and conflicting than intellectual ones. We should, however, listen more and more to these instinctive signals as they may well be the key to the richness of ethical complexity so vital to informed moral decision making.

Dewey was an early and avid champion of the work of Charles Darwin. As a result of this he was always concerned to see his philosophy as a growing organic reality with an inner life of its own. Just as there are many aspects of our biological life which we do not fully understand or advert to at all, and yet they contribute to our growth and development, so new and unsuspected aspects of ethics constantly appear. It is useful to try to seek out the genetic origins of these ideas. Just as the more we know the genetic bases of human, or any, biology the more we may come to understand the product of these factors, so there may be a few central ethical impulses or drives which are key to each one of us and to all of us collectively. These drives will be impulsive and emotive. There will also be a considerable number of them. They will not always be in harmony with each other. Conflict is the very essence of life. (In the next chapter contemporary developments of this genetic theme will be explored in the ethical approaches associated with sociobiology.)

It will be useful to come to realize as much as possible the functionings individually and collectively of these inner possibilities. One or another passion or interest may seem to be and may well in fact be self-serving. Others may appear more altruistic. A check on the direction of these drives might be the perceived consequences of working one or another of them to the advantage or expense of others. There is a strong spatial and temporal dimension to the playing out of inner emotive impulses. There is a time and place when they can be effectively deployed and when they can not.[22]

The diagnostic and prognostic practice of medicine is a salient model case of genetic development. Health and disease have each their own inner course of progress or decay. Medicine intervenes at only a certain time and place. The art or craft nature of medicine dictates that as much as possible we do not impose a final solution but try to get in harmony with the biological and psychological rhythms we are encountering. The biological and psychological rhythms of the health care professional interact in integral ways with the biological and psychological rhythms of the patient. Creative conflicts abound.

As a consequence we cannot look to any neat and completed theory, medical or ethical, for the solution to problematic cases.

Rather there is a need to have theory grow in the midst of practice. Dewey is really reversing the distinction between theoretical and applied ethics. Then and now applied ethics is down played as being a second rate kind of operation with little intellectual strength and coherence. Dewey would say that theoretical ethical systems are empty and vapid. The only real ethics is the pragmatic working with uncertainty. We must be attuned to the complexity of the particular, the challenge of change and novelty, the accidental character of things.[23]

We feel within ourselves often strong propensities to one or another sort of action. Sometimes it is correct to follow these instincts, sometimes not. A basically useful deployment of our energies over a long period of time marks the virtuous individual. Long term catering to debilitating tendencies marks vice.[24] One of the fundamental entrance points into ethics is the point at which we question the patternings of virtue or vice.[25]

One of the greatest problem areas in medical practice has to do with the stance a physician should take when dealing with a patient who is trapped by a habit deleterious to that individual's health. Are we to be highly aggressive in trying to get the smoker to stop? Should we demand that our patients lose weight? How serious a situation is alcohol abuse? Should homosexuals be lectured so as not to contract AIDS?

What about the habits and patterns of physicians? Do we not all tend at some time or another to fall into certain types of diagnoses and prognoses which blind us to problems and possibilities? Have we adapted a certain way of dealing with patients which we apply pretty much across the board with not enough attention to personal differences?

What happens when the habitual behavior patterns of physicians and patients come into sometimes radical conflict? Are we primarily just at the service of the patient's wishes or do we have any kind of obligation to try to better the patient as we see the need for help and intervention?

In all of this it is important to remember that whatever course of action we may decide to take, we should not ever attempt a total solution to the situation. Rather the ethical question is related to just what small action we should take at what time and place in order to bring about the best practical solution.[26]

Sometimes in an effort to try to accomplish too much at once physicians can make moral blunders. For example, Joe's family physician, Dr. Raymond, works at Memorial Hospital as an attending doctor. He knows Joe is addicted to heroin and he has several times tried to convince Joe to seek help.

Recently Joe went to see Dr. Raymond for his yearly physical and the physician noticed Joe's physical condition was deteriorating. Dr. Raymond was aware that Joe's wife did not know about his habit and that Joe had managed to carry out most of his responsibilities reasonably well. So there was little external pressure on Joe to get help.

Dr. Raymond believed that it was his obligation as a physician to help Joe but he also believed he had an obligation to protect Joe's privacy. Unfortunately the results of Joe's most recent check-up convinced Dr. Raymond that it was his duty to do more than just lecture his patient, so he informed Joe's wife of the problem.

Physicians have to recognize their limits as well as their duties. They not only have limits to their skill, but they also have limits to their authority and may make the already complex problems of medical practice even more intractable.

Every moral situation involves problematic questions of who is in the right and wrong. If we firmly believe that we are right and the other person wrong, this may be a clue to our abandoning of ethical complexity and tact.[27] The most righteous people are regularly the most unethical.

In an attempt to clarify just how we work through problematic ethical situations, Dewey points out that there are three factors in the decision making process. First, there must be a certain amount of quite clear knowledge. Second, there must be a strong and firm decision. Special to this decision is the felt sense that one is clearly and precisely choosing a particular course of action. This means that one is especially attentive to the act of choosing itself. Third, these decisions should arise out of and be in the context of a strong and stable character.[28]

These three elements in decision making have a rather special application in modern medical practice. Now more than ever there is a stress on clear and comprehensive knowledge in medicine. The rapid expansion of technology and research has made the task of providing an adequate medical education almost impossible. Students regularly have the experience of being tossed from one service to another so rapidly that they have little time to really comprehend what is going on. Often the experience is rather the realization of just how little they know. The whole situation can breed more of a lack of confidence than an understanding of medicine. The result is often that there is a drive to stay within the confines of a quite narrow specialty and even to concentrate on only one part of that specialty. That specialty, at least, can be mastered and so provide the proper knowledge base for clear decision. Even the field of family practice, which would be the most general field in medicine, is treated more and more as a specialty in its own right with an ever growing body of knowledge required.

Even more problematic is the voluntary character of decision making. It might seem at first that any decision would automatically have to be voluntary, but Dewey is concerned to point out to us that there should be a strong commitment to the decided upon act to make the intervention truly effective. Given the extremes of levels of knowledge in medicine, what regularly happens is a sort of voluntaristic drift. Rather than clearly and decisively taking action in a case, we let things drift for considerable periods of time. The more technology available the more this can go on. There is so much data provided and so many aspects of the case to be considered that we can dawdle on them for long periods. The wealth of information can provide a good excuse for not taking action and we let things sort themselves out. This is especially the case in many a termination of life situation. Often clear and decisive action should have been taken at an earlier or critical juncture rather than let things drag on. The longer the voluntaristic procrastination the more difficult any decisive action will become.

The right blend of knowledge and decision occurs when a habitual tendency to take decisive action has been built up over a long period of time. This is what is meant by the third factor of character in decision making. Since medicine is the practice of a pragmatic art we do not have the luxury of living only or primarily in the world of knowledge. Rather intervention and action are the essence of medical practice. A habitual readiness to take prompt and precise action will characterize a helpful and effective physician. Only the careful and constant taking of action will make us feel at ease in making action and decision the center of medical practice. Medicine is no place for the timorous or timid as the following case will show.

Mr. D. was admitted to Memorial Hospital on a Monday afternoon to be prepared for an operation to remove an abdominal aneurysm. He had a history of heart trouble including two myocardial infarctions, one in 1960 and the other in 1968, and recent attacks of angina. His stepdaughter also reported that he had apparently suffered a mild stroke for which he had not sought treatment the previous summer.

Mr. D.'s second wife had died nearly a year earlier from a sudden and quite unexpected MCI and since then he had been extremely depressed and exhibited erratic behavior. A routine check-up at another hospital, larger and better equipped than Memorial but further from his home, had uncovered the aneurysm. The physician there recommended surgical removal of the aneurysm followed by insertion of a pacemaker to help regulate his heartbeat. Mr. D. decided to have the surgery performed at Memorial because it was closer to his home than the other hospital.

After Mr. D. settled into the ICU the night before surgery his son and daughter indicated to the ICU nurse that he would like to have a Do Not Resuscitate order placed in the chart. But the ICU nurse did not want to comply and Mr. D.'s children were reluctant to press the issue or discuss it in more detail with their father.

The operation was successful but afterwards Mr. D.'s angina increased. The attending physician ordered nitroglycerin patches for him but was convinced that Mr. D. would leave the ICU in a few days. There was no cardiologist on staff and no one took the initiative to bring in one from another hospital. The son and daughter went back to their homes and there was no further discussion of a DNR order.

Two days later Mr. D., who had continued to have intermittent angina attacks, suffered an MCI with his heart stopping for about nine minutes. He was resuscitated and placed on a ventilator but he was comatose. The children returned to the hospital immediately even though they lived a considerable distance away and asked that the ventilator be removed since Mr. D. had often expressed a desire not to be kept alive by "extraordinary means". Three days later Mr. D. was weaned from the ventilator until he could breathe on his own. The neurologist had determined that he would never recover cortical functioning. He continued to breathe in an otherwise vegetative state for four weeks.

There are several points in this story where it is clear that procrastination on the part of the attending physician, the nurses and Mr. D.'s children prevented a decision from being made that could have resulted in Mr. D. undergoing a more dignified dying process or might perhaps have even saved his life. If you were the attending physician, the nurse or one of Mr. D.'s children, what would you have done? Was there a need here for some sort of moral development on the part of many of the' people involved in this case?

Dewey also here anticipates the whole contemporary stress on moral development. He notes that a good character must be worked on over a considerable period of time. There are stages in that development. Key to those stages for Dewey is the amount of decisive commitment we can bring to our choices. He clearly favors the active and involved type of personality.[29] While Dewey does not make explicit that he thinks that it is less dangerous to be active than inactive, this could be construed from his presentation. In terms of medical practice it might be right to go along with this in that an as informed as possible intervention does bring the situation under our control more than little or no intervention. The ancient medical ethical dictum of "do no harm" should not be taken primarily to mean "take no or little action." Rather it would emphasize acting in a competent and decisive fashion.

This kind of decisive action over a period of time will penetrate deep into the make-up of our desires, intents, choices and dispositions.[30] There will be a very strong influence on the way in which we experience our basic outlook on reality. Dewey's pragmatism is here in great strength. The strong, actively involved individual is perceived as the most satisfied and effective person. People go into medicine in order to accomplish great things. Dewey says that we will develop the character of being effective physicians by daringly and deeply acting.

A very useful distinction is made between standards and purposes, aims, or ends-in-view. Standards look to the past, ends-in-view to the future. It is important in decision making and the habits formed in this progress to set our sights on aims or ends-in-view. If we are always or primarily concerned to be satisfying standards, we will never be actually able to do this as the standards are always changing. If the habitual practice of virtue is taken to be some type or other of standard behavior we will never be satisfied in our pursuit of virtue as we will never feel that we have reached that ideal standard.[31]

In medicine this would mean that the attempt to adhere to just standard medical practice would doom one to mediocrity. The challenge of medicine is always to go beyond what is now known and done. Even the most common family practitioner must be always searching for and trying out new and better procedures. Medicine is an area of high goals and aims which have barely begun to be fulfilled and realized. The virtuous physician is the adventurous physician.

The present malpractice crisis has cast a certain tone to this pursuit of excellence. Since negligence in medical practice means falling below the level of practice and competence of one's peers, there is more of a push to just adhere to the standards and not be too adventuresome. But this tendency should be resisted. Going beyond the standards to something better is not against the notion of standard medical practice. In fact one of the key elements of standard medical practice is to be constantly seeking and employing newer and better techniques. One way of falling below the level of standard medical practice is to not be aggressive in new medicine. Standing still here means to quickly fall behind.

Because standards look to the past they are useful in assessing the strong actions that we have already taken. The individual who habitually takes clear and strong action will find not only personal satisfaction but the approbation and support of peers and dependants. Strong, decisive, informed intervention wins admiration and emulation. But if we aim too directly at this group affirmation and approbation we will not be inclined to take the only kinds of actions which can bring this to us.[32]

In this pragmatic context Dewey has situated the older notion of friendship and support as so critical to the habitual practice of virtue ethics as this was first mapped out by Aristotle. Proper decisive activity will bring about the kind of mutual teamwork and support so essential as the proper social context for personal achievement and success. Any member of a medical team knows at once this theory works well in actual cooperative group practice.

One massive segment of the medical team is now, however, finding considerable difficulty in being able to practice beyond its level of standards so as to achieve excellence. Nurses find that physicians and administrators often want to keep them confined to a certain level of practice. It is difficult to feel comfortable in taking the initiative. This contributes in great part to the malaise in nursing today. They too must be seen as an integral part of the team which can and must make constant constructive contribution to medical progress. The virtuous habitual practice of technical friendship must extend wide. Consider the role of the nurses in the following case.

Jerry is a 28-year-old white male who was recently admitted to Memorial Hospital for treatment of pneumonia. He is profoundly mentally retarded and has cerebral palsy as a consequence of an intracranial hemorrage at birth. He also has hemophilia A and was found to be HIV positive two years ago. Most of his recent hospitalizations have been related to bleeding secondary to his hemophliac status. Jerry, although mentally retarded, is capable of crude communication and is able to demonstrate preferences in regard to care givers, play objects and food. He can crawl and feed himself but otherwise is completely dependent on others. He was raised at home by his mother with whom he has a close relationship.

A diagnosis of pneumocystis carinii pneumonia (PCP) was made and he was placed on bactrim for treatment by his attending physician, Dr. Jones. His hospital course was complicated by frequent respiratory distress, fevers, an inguinal hemotoma secondary to a femoral venipuncture and apneic episodes. Jerry's mother stayed with him during the entire two week hospitalization except for the last two days of treatment. She showed an enormous concern for her son during each crisis and insisted on aggressive therapy at all times. During rounds Dr. Jones indicated to residents and nurses that he felt that he did not approve of Jerry's mother's decisions concerning treatment and he also appeared agitated about Jerry's very poor prognosis.

Eventually Jerry improved and plans were made for discharge. His reaction to bactrim indicated that his pneumonia was most likely PCP and represented his first HIV positive related illness. On the day prior to discharge he was given aerosolized pentamadine which is currently the prophylactic treatment of choice for AIDS-related PCP. Many patients at Memorial receive aerosolized pentamadine on a monthly basis for prophylactic treatment, but because of Jerry's physical and mental status in addition to being a hemophiliac with AIDS a decision was made not to administer pentamadine on a regular basis. The mother was not informed of this decision nor was she told the value of a treatment with pentamadine. Jerry was to be followed up at Memorial whenever symptoms recurred.

The two nurses who had spent a great deal of time caring for Jerry and discussing his condition with his mother were put off by the decision not to prescribe pentamadine. But they were even more concerned by Dr. Jones' refusal to inform Jerry's mother of the decision without telling her of the recent studies documenting the treatment's value. Each of them confronted Dr. Jones separately about their concerns. In both instances he told them he was the doctor and that they should say absolutely nothing about penta-madine to Jerry's mother. Communal trust and support here seem sadly lacking.

The communal and supportive social aspects of virtue will be experienced and fostered if we each individually put into practice certain key characteristics of virtue. Dewey thinks that the practice of virtue must be wholehearted, sincere, continuous, persistent, impartial.[33] There must also be a stressing or balancing of certain virtues against and in harmony with other virtues. The pursuit of a single virtue in isolation will distort the complexity of the situation. It might make us fall back on the adhering to a standard rather than the flexibility required to pursue ends-in-view. Dewey thinks it is useful to balance pragmatically such things as the old basic cardinal virtues of prudence, justice, courage and temperance. But he thinks that what holds all of the virtues together is love.[34] Love is the drive to go always beyond the merely required to the better and best that we can accomplish. It is the ultimate pursuit of excellence. The more we aim at high goals the more we win the love and support of those around us. The practice of medicine is the practice of love. What real reason is there to stay in it if we do not love our patients? Money and prestige and affirmation in themselves are standards which will never ultimately satisfy us. The pursuit of them for their own sake is futile. The satisfaction in medicine is found in the love for the work that we do in that this work precisely and conscientiously done manifests in a helpful and concrete way the love we have for other human beings. The pursuit of the highest aim brings the highest support and satisfaction.

There are at least two situations in which habit fails. One would be the time at which we have not as yet really formulated the basis of a habitual commitment to a certain type or course of action. The other would occur when for a variety of reasons a certain type of habitual behavior must be changed or modified.

In these kinds of situations Dewey says that we must have recourse to a kind of reflection so as to again build up proper habitual behavior patterns. The purpose of reflection is the setting up again of rather clear ends-in-view. But we often experience a difficulty about this in that it becomes problematic as to just what our ends or goals in a particular case should be. There may seem to be a conflict between short and long term goals. The short term goals are more governed or set by immediately felt drives or impulses. We feel often a desperate need to do something, to become actively involved. Long term goals require more aloofness from the pressure of the situation. They respond much more to rational rather than impulsive behavior.[35] Dewey favors the rational approach. We ought to clearly and reasonably set our goals. But he is also concerned to make sure that this rational analysis caters as much as possible to the impulses and desires which press upon us in the heat of a problem.[36] In this he states in a modern way the concern already noted in Aquinas to blend emotional and rational experiences in a morally sound prudential judgment.

In the practice of medicine critical and unexpected cases often force major reconsideration. We may find in the treatment of a terminally ill patient that we are not sure of the relation of our short term goals to our long term ones. We strongly feel that something now must be done in order at least to alleviate suffering, but we are not sure how to fit these interventions into long term prognosis. Are we in fact actually prolonging a physical and emotional agony which we would be much better advised to end?

In these sorts of cases the strong temptation is to cater to felt needs and impulses. This is fortified and abetted by the many medical anomalies and uncertainties which such a case can present. Rather than really work out a clearly articulated long range plan, the exigencies and minutiae of day to day care dominate. We are in a sort of medical and ethical drift. Demands, often highly emotive, from other members of the health care team press us to cater most to present problems.

Development and deployment of a clear long range plan requires a considerable amount of moral courage. This is true of any major ethical decision. The more ethical theory that can be brought to bear the better. This is a time for reason and rationality. But it is vital that any long range plan also cater as much as possible to present concerns. Again it is most important that an attending physician understand and empathize with the feelings and points of view of patients, families and other members of the health care team. Especially important here is the integration of nursing and social work staff into the larger picture in a collaborative and supportive way.

The case of suicidal Henry who is HIV positive discussed earlier in this chapter provides a good example of how a collaborative effort can yield a treatment plan that is more sensitive to the needs of patients and their loved ones than might be accomplished by physicians alone.

Henry, the 36-year-old artist who had severely incapacitated himself by attempting suicide, had been a subject of concern for the social worker, the speech pathologist, nurses, attending physician, infectious disease fellow and ethics consultant. The social worker had found a nursing home that admits HIV infected persons. This is very rare within Memorial's catchment area.

The ethics consultant asked a student enrolled in a humanities elective to get involved in the case as his course project. The student spent some time with Henry and very creatively suggested that a speech pathologist might test Henry to determine if he could communicate in any way. In fact Henry did manage to communicate, though in a very rudimentary manner, that he did not want to remain in the hospital or go to a nursing home. He wanted to return to his own home and receive the minimal care necessary to sustain his life.

Several conferences in addition to the one described above took place over a period of two weeks. At all of these conferences the nurses were able to add significant information about Henry's level of functions because they interacted with him every afternoon. As a result of these conferences the physician was persuaded to avoid making any hasty decisions and Tom, Henry's roommate and guardian, changed his mind about pressing to have all his life support systems removed. Henry went home in a situation of much more clarity as regards both short and long term goals on the part of all those involved in the case.

Experimental medicine presents a particularly problematic potential conflict between long and short range goals. This becomes most critical in cases of experimentation on terminally ill patients. Even though these patients and their families know when they sign often elaborate consent forms that the actual benefit they may experience from experimental therapy is slight, as the treatment proceeds it is difficult to not experience false hopes. After all, a large number of the most competent people in the hospital are now working on you. There may be an impressive use of complex technology. One may be hooked up to elaborate machines which seem very busy in making noises of intriguing kinds and producing bafflingly enticing readouts.

But the goal of all of this is often not very much the cure of the patient, but rather the advancement of medical science. Rare indeed is the terminal patient who sees scientific advance as the basic reason for entering an experimental protocol. Even a person trying as hard as possible to be an ultimate altruist slips into some sort of self-serving in the face of death.

The rigidity of the research protocol further constrains both physician and patient. Not only might certain more immediately palliative maneuvers be ruled out by the medical limits to the experimentation, but often even more extraneous forces impinge. Since almost all research is either government or private interest funded, finance dictates greatly the setting of long range goals. The balance between short term impulses to cure or care and the requirements of the larger general protocol can become intense indeed as the next case illustrates.

Mrs. R. was brought into the emergency room at 1.45 a.m. She had been in an automobile accident. She suffered from severe shock due to head injury, major abrasions on her arms and legs, open wounds on her face, neck and shoulders, and was bleeding profusely. She was 63 and all efforts to reach her family had been futile. It was later learned that her husband was on vacation and they had no children.

The resident on duty that night, Dr. P., knew the trauma procedures thoroughly but he also knew that they entailed risks as well as benefits. Furthermore, Memorial Hospital had several trauma-related research programs underway and Dr. P. knew that he had a responsibility to put as many new patients on the protocols as possible. Mrs. R. was a suitable subject for one of the experiments but the drug being tested in that experiment was already known to have side effects. Nonetheless, the experiment had already suggested that the drug was efficacious in restoring some degree of functioning to patients in shock.

Whatever Dr. P. decided to do for Mrs. R. would involve a violation of some moral principles. If he did nothing until she or a surrogate could provide adequately informed consent, Mrs. R. might be much worse off than when she was brought in because she was hemorrhaging. If he used the standard procedures and drugs to ameliorate shock she might get better but the experiment would suffer and she might be deprived of a more efficacious drug than the standard treatment. But she would also be protected from some of the possible risks of the new drug about which not enough was known to help in making this decision.

He had to make a decision in a hurry and he decided that Mrs. R.'s right to participate in the decision that she be put on the experimental protocol outweighed both the uncertain benefits of the new drug and the overall utility the experiment was likely to yield. So he treated her in the standard manner with the aim in view of relieving her shock as safely as possible.

An attempt to map out the ethics of such conflict laden contexts in terms of patient rights and physician duties can become so problematic as to be counterproductive. Dewey suggests that a better way to envision the ethics of this kind of encounter is to build the various dynamics of human interaction into a larger view of ends and purposes. We must be aware as much as possible of the complexities both rational and emotional which come into play. But he has an ever abiding optimistic faith in the ability of people to be sensitive to each other in a cooperative way.[37] This is so because he always emphasizes the social context of the development and practice of virtue.

In the course of the human working through of problematic ethical cases there are built up a set of principles and rules. Principles tend to be more abstract and intellectual, rules more practical and pragmatic.[38] Principles would seem to be more concerned with the formulation of ends-in-view, rules more with the following of more immediate impulses. Dewey would like an organic interplay between the two, but he is here very cautious about the over-reliance on principles. If they are not fitted to the situations out of which they originally grew, they become stringent laws unto themselves. When this happens Dewey thinks that we end up having to serve the principles rather than having the principles serve us. The attempt to mitigate these harsh and unyielding principles is casuistry. Dewey has rather harsh words about this type of moral endeavor as he thinks that it tends to break up the holistic moral experience into little compartments or pigeonholes.[39] This makes us follow too closely the letter of the law. We also then set up a highly legalistic system of rewards and punishments. All of this may destroy the sense of freedom and responsibility so central to the moral and ethical experience.[40]

We must always remember that moral principle is a tool to be used in working out the difficulties of a particular problem. There is no move to do away with these principles, but rather to make them an integral part of the ethical project. Rather than providing the final answer they should suggest ways of acting. They should provide us with a proper point of view in coming at a problem.[41] The kinds of principles put forward in recent codes of ethics by various types of medical groups tend currently to follow Dewey's monition more than not.

In our attempt to incorporate moral principles into our everyday ethics Dewey asks us to look especially to four rich sources.[42] It is important to considerably study the codes of ethics produced at various times by conscientious groups. An understanding of the reasons why these codes were formulated and of the conflicts in and among codes will provide a great deal of material not only for ethical reflection but also for practical use. More and more as medical ethics becomes a separate study and discipline of its own this kind of work is being done, and it has been yielding very practical results.

We should also consider legal history, juridical decisions and legislative activity. While law is not the same as ethics and so operates on its own set of principles and practice, there is so much interplay and influence of one on the other that much can be gained from exploring the mechanisms of the other. The main reason for studying law from an ethical point of view is the window it gives us on the human mind and spirit struggling with problematic situations. While the methodologies of law and ethics may differ they are both trying to reach often the same goals.

Dewey is very strong on building the latest findings of science into any ethical enquiry. He stresses the role of the sciences which are more closely concerned with human matters such as biology, physiology, medicine, psychology and psychiatry. The social nature of the human project must also be looked into in a study of sociology, economics and politics.

A keen and exhaustive study of history can show in considerable detail the modalities of human striving which are so central to the ethical enterprise. Reading and employment of biographical materials might serve the same purpose.

There is clearly in John Dewey's pragmatism a strong sense of the need to incorporate biological, psychological and social factors into any building up of a habit or virtue approach to ethics. A final chapter will survey in considerable detail these factors and others in an attempt to map out how a virtue ethic might be made most current and contemporary as a potent tool in the solution of moral questions.

6

CONTEMPORARY DEVELOPMENTS IN VIRTUE ETHICS

Just as the Aristotelian development of virtue ethics worked in a framework of human activity considered as part of an organic biological whole, so there is a significant aspect of the present discussion of virtue ethics which should be situated in terms of some recent developments in biological theory. While a number of the authors to be cited do not so explicitly deal with an ethics of virtue as such, the kinds of ethical approach taken are in many ways compatible with this ethical point of view. This is most important in the field of medical ethics where biology permeates all ethical decision making.

A key article in the *Journal of the American Medical Association* is very critical of the majority of current medical ethical writing. The authors think that there is far too much concentration on questions of patients' rights and physicians' duties. Rather there is needed a more integral ethics which can situate values in the biologically based rhythms of birth, growth and development, of life and death. Appeal is made to the grand tradition of teleological ethics represented by such figures as Aristotle, Darwin, James and the founder of sociobiology, Edward O. Wilson.[1] The same authors in a lead editorial in the *Archives of Internal Medicine* term this a biopsychosocial approach.[2] The human condition is one in which these three elements are constantly at work in a kind of harmonic unity. Ethical activity is an almost musical blending of these various factors in an ever creative revelation of possibilities for goodness, growth and development. The weighing and balancing of possible procedures so central to virtue ethics makes the biopsychosocial approach its natural home.

THE BIOLOGICAL FRAME

Charles Darwin was a man who in many fundamental ways was deeply disturbed and upset by his own scientific findings. He was born into a very well established British family and lived out his life during the highly orderly days of Victorian England. He liked to have everything in its proper place. Any hint of disorder could lead to the sort of chaotic conditions which the British Empire took great pains to eradicate as much as possible from the face of the earth. Knowledge, self-control and a certain reserve would be the ways to bring about the order so needed in human affairs.

Having finished theological studies at Cambridge University, young Charles Darwin embarked on a voyage around the coast of South America. The purpose of this British government expedition was the mapping out of the parts of the South American continent. Darwin was along somewhat for the ride but with the encouragement to collect and catalog as many specimens of botanical and biological life as he might find of use and interest. His discoveries led him eventually to conclusions both as to the great age of many of the fossils which he uncovered and to the realization that an organic chain of development linked one species of fossil to another until their descendants arrived to live and die on the earth as we know and find it now. But Darwin realized that biological life as we now find it is very much the product of a multitude of quite chance biological encounters at the whim of the vagaries of time and place.

There was a further problem. All the evidence which Darwin amassed for his theory of evolution was grossly anatomical or phenotypical. He knew that there had to be some inner biological mechanism deeply microscopic which would explain variations within a species and the possibility of a development of one species from another. But he personally had no scientific evidence for these genotypic procedures. When, in the early 1950s at Darwin's home university of Cambridge, Watson and Crick discovered the structure of DNA the missing link in Darwin's theory was in place. There is now a clear way of understanding the interplay between phenotype and genotype, but a new and desperate problem arises for ethics. Is this interplay a matter primarily or basically of chance encounter or is there a deeper underlying order and harmony which we can discover in the biological bases of our existence? Depending on the answer we would have to see the psychological and social experiences which are so rooted in our biology as being either random and chaotic or ordered and rational. Only if we find some sort of ordering will we have a biopsychosocial life form capable of nourishing a virtue ethic.

One of the most sustained attempts to find order in this situation of possible chaos is the work of Edward O. Wilson, the founder of a vast synthetic approach to the problem of the inner harmonies of the human situation. The approach is called sociobiology. The project had some rather unusual beginnings. Wilson's first major work is a vast and detailed study of insect society. But a number of very important ethical considerations emerged from this study. Wilson observed that a number of insect societies are extremely altruistic. This means that the individual insect experiences life as part of a larger social scheme to which individual contribution even to the sacrifice of one's life is necessary for the life, growth and development of the colony.[3] The reason for this kind of perhaps primitive ethical behavior is in the genetic inheritance of each insect. Each is programmed to play a part in the larger social picture. The individual appears to be a function of society rather than the other way around. But this is not to deny the importance of the individual for without the individual society itself is obviously impossible.

In the insect societies these functions are regularly hierarchically organized with lower members of society serving in often self-sacrificing ways those higher. But those members of insect society who are seemingly higher up on the ladder are really only there because they serve a crucial function in the life of the whole insect colony. The queen bee, ant or termite has her high status because of the central life giving role she performs. Insects at the top of the hierarchy are in this way altruists of a very special sort. There is something profoundly ethical sounding in all of this analysis. And it is ethics of the most penetrating sort in that the kinds of self-sacrificing altruism found in insect societies look suspiciously close to some of the highest ideals of animal or human society. We tend to call this kind of extreme altruistic behavior dedicated and self-effacing love, the highest ideal of ethics.

Not only as regards altruism does Wilson find similarities between animal and insect behavior. The structures of kinship will also play, for instance, a key role. These structures will take a dramatically different turn in animal society. Here there is much more clearly the emergence of the individual. An individual animal appears to have much more of a set of distinguishable personal traits than an individual insect. Any one of us who has lived for any time with a dog or a cat knows that each one of them has a certain approach to life which looks very much like a somewhat personal set of character traits. Any competent animal breeder will also be able to tell you that at least to some extent these traits are genetically inherited. As you go about training your dog or cat, you are also aware that these traits are also heavily culturally conditioned. There is a rich but problematic interplay between genes and culture. Somehow the inner harmonies which are the very stuff of virtue ethics must take into account both factors.

Wilson in the very last paragraph of *The Insect Societies* holds out the promise that the study of the principles of behavioral and population biology will point us in the direction of being able to develop an overarching understanding of social patterns common to both insects and animals.[4] Also here some of the basic methodologies of sociobiology are already clearly in place. There is a concentration on social issues as those of most importance in understanding any grouping of insects or animals. But all social matters are radically grounded in biology. Biology is the key to sociology. So there is a kind of reduction of social concerns to biological data. Within the realm of biology itself larger biological structures can only be understood in terms of the smaller genetic mechanisms which produce and foster those larger structures. Put technically, phenotypes must be understood in terms of genotypes. There is even something of a reduction of phenotype to genotype.

While these patterns of sociobiology are rather clear in *The Insect Societies* Wilson is quite careful not to include speculations about human behavior in this early study. He will not be so reticent at all in the next major work which he produced.

Sociobiology: the New Synthesis studies in great detail the social behavior of animals as well as insects. There is also a most provocative final chapter applying the results of these studies to human behavior. The book's opening chapter on the morality of the gene clearly sets up this whole project as of enormous ethical significance. Wilson is convinced that the root and springs of our ethical behavior are genetic. Genes are concerned to insure their own reproductive survival. As a result the phenotypical products of genetic programming must engage in behavior which will be an efficient mixture of mechanisms of personal survival, reproduction and altruism. But because phenotypes are programmed to do this by their hidden genes, their overt surface behavior becomes ethically ambivalent whenever there is a threat to these three key factors. There is a joining of love and hate, aggression and fear, expansiveness and withdrawal in blends designed not to promote the happiness and survival of the individual, but rather the maximum transmission of the controlling genes.[5] At the human, and to probably a lesser extent at the animal level, this means that our conscious surface ethical behavior is at the service of our unconscious drives. These drives are in turn securely rooted in the genetic necessities of reproduction and survival.

The animal groups with whom we most share conscious and unconscious ethical traits are the higher primates. We are, of course, genetically closely related. *Sociobiology's* final chapter provided an exhaustive listing of socially ethical traits which we share with primates. Some are shared with only certain other primates: group size, group cohesiveness, openness of the group to other groups, involvement of the male in parental care, intensity and forms of territorial defense. Some are shared with almost all other primates: aggressive male dominance systems, scaling of responses in aggressive interactions, prolonged maternal care, prolonged socialization of young, matrilineal organization. There are some socially ethical traits peculiar to humans: true language, elaborate culture, sexual activity continuous through the menstrual cycle, formalized incest taboos, marriage exchange rules, kinship networks, cooperative division of labor between adult males and females.[6]

Ethical behavior at practically all levels comes in for a quite revisionist reading in this approach. But the whole project remains securely in the framework of understanding of the human situation as being one of an interweaving of elements of body and soul, mind and matter which has its roots especially in Aristotle and its development in Thomas Aquinas. In the latter, for instance, two of the cardinal virtues, fortitude and temperance, are associated with respectively the basic bodily drives of aggression and concupiscence. The other two cardinal virtues, justice and prudence, are more mentally oriented. While neither Aristotle nor Aquinas have any clear notion of an unconscious, fortitude and temperance are more concerned with areas now considered to be either intimately connected to or fundamentally rooted in the unconscious. The other two cardinal virtues can be seen as trying to cater to the demands and drives of the unconscious.

The specifically ethical consequences of sociobiological theory were explored by Wilson in the popularization of his theories in the book which won him the Pulitzer Prize, *On Human Nature*. Here the dichotomy between conscious surface behavior and depth unconscious behavior is even more clearly drawn. More clearly thought out or rational activity is associated with surface conscious behavior; more emotive irrational activity is associated with depth unconscious behavior. Genetic activity is so deeply rooted as the source of our conscious life that we find ourselves for the most part in the situation of responding to the signals which our genes send to the surface from the richness of our more emotive unconscious. As a result Wilson thinks that the most important events and decisions in our life are and should be emotive ones. The most important ethical decisions should be felt to be the correct ones, not so much known to be so.[7]

Also in this text there is a precise treatment of the problem of aggression and altruism. The question has genetic roots. If phenotypes are basically vehicles for genetic enhancement and survival, then genes seem to be very selfish and manipulative of their environment. This selfishness is consciously carried out in human behavior patterns of a drive to aggressive advancement. Wilson is concerned to show that these aggressive patterns are also at one and the same time altruistic. He does this by suggesting a distinction between hard-core and soft-core altruism.[8] Hard-core altruism would mean action taken with very little or no thought of personal reward or remuneration whatever. Wilson thinks that this seldom or ever occurs. Soft-core altruism is a genuine care and concern for others but with the hope and expectation of personal reward and satisfaction.

Seen from a gene's point of view soft-core altruism makes a good deal of sense. To survive and thrive the gene must produce a phenotype congenial to it. The gene must be at the genuine service of the phenotype. It must really want to altruistically enhance the life and the health of the phenotype. But there is then the reward of enhanced genetic health and reproduction. Since in sociobiology all social behavior, including human social behavior, must be understood in terms of genetic propensities, we find ourselves most regularly involved in socially altruistic behavior. Individual members of the socially organic groupings that form human culture must be self-sacrificing altruists in order not primarily that the group will survive and thrive but that the individual will do so. This altruism is quite soft-core, but it is altruism.

There are very few physicians who are not altruists. Often they like to think of themselves or have others think of them as being hard-core altruists. And in many ways they have a proper claim on this title. There is a certain mystique about the practice of medicine which drives many physicians to be as self-sacrificing as possible, regularly working themselves to a state of emotional and physical exhaustion. Part of the reason for this must lie in the perceived needs of people who come to them for help. One of the most dramatic examples of this which I have ever encountered was the response of a young highly trained M.D., Ph.D. clinical oncology fellow to my question as to why she would choose to work so closely with suffering terminal cancer patients. "They need me the most," she said.

Not only is there the individual drive to be heroically altruistic in the practice of medicine, but the profession itself demands this kind of dedication from its members. While time and again there are calls, for instance, for reform in the killing schedules imposed on interns and residents, it is felt that somehow everyone has to go through this experience in order to be a good doctor. But does this hard-core altruism have a soft-core base?

Medicine, even with the contemporary controversies surrounding it, is still a profession of immense prestige. While physicians work very hard indeed to attain the position of respect they find themselves in, they also expect to receive this respect and are quite upset when it is not shown. Patients have their place and should keep it. Older and wiser physicians are not under any circumstances to be contradicted. Many a patient's treatment protocol has been dictated as much by the hierarchies of physician power structures as by the best treatment options in the case. In order to satisfy the emotively felt aggressive drives one feels in being a physician altruistic social behavior is mandatory. One must be altruistic to patients and to colleagues. It is genuine altruism but soft-core and practiced in the sociobiological context of hierarchical power structures.

In Memorial Hospital, like many other teaching hospitals, the hierarchy of the health care team has the following structure:

attending physician
resident

head nurse
intern
staff nurses
medical student

This structure often leaves the medical students, staff nurses and interns feeling overworked and oppressed. But people at the higher end of the hierarchy sometimes understand that it is in their enlightened self-interest to step out of role and help relieve some of the pressure on those at the bottom of the hierarchy.

Bob Jeffries is an internal medicine attending and his wife, Mary, is a head nurse at Memorial. Partly for this reason, Dr. Jeffries is somewhat more sensitive to the nursing shortage. One night, he was on call when a 78-year-old man was brought into the Intensive Care Unit with a myocardial infarction. The ICU was short staffed that night, and two nurses were working double shifts. While Dr. Jeffries struggled to stabilize the patient, he noticed that the ICU was full and that the nurses could not handle the load by themselves.

Normally Dr. Jeffries would not consider it his job to help take vital signs, change IV bags, etc. But this was clearly not a normal situation. One of the nurses, on her second shift of the day, looked exhausted and had become short-tempered. So Dr. Jeffries offered to take her place for a half hour, while she went on break. Observing the traditional hierarchy, however gratifying to his ego, would not in this situation be in the best interests of the patients in the ICU, nor would it have been in the best interests of the health care team.

How would you have acted in this kind of situation? Was Dr. Jeffries acting prudently, given the possibility that he might have been called to another emergency while the nurse was still on break?

Wilson is much criticised for his reductionism. This entails the reduction of social units through larger biological units to genetic components as well as the concentration on individual genetic units or genes. He has taken these criticisms very seriously and tried to reply to them in a co-authored book with Charles J. Lumsden called *Genes, Mind and Culture*. To concentrate on the second problem first, the authors note that no gene acts alone in and of itself but that there is rather a number of operations which a single gene or group of genes performs in units. A single gene in the

DNA strand often, for instance, has many functions. Also the reading off or spinning out of RNA from DNA on the road to the building up of the basic proteins is a cooperative activity building up biological complexes which in turn build up social complexes. The whole of the human experience is one of the networking of the various configurations. The biological and social networks are governed by in-built rules which build and then guide and direct their activities. Wilson terms these epigenetic rules. The nature of these rules is to weave and unweave ever more complex and changing biological and social patterns. The stress is on the richly complex possibilities of the patternings rather than on the individual pieces of a single pattern.[9] Aristotle's dream of an inner ordering of teleology running through all forms of biological and social life forms has found a rather startling modern advocate.

The epigenetic rules run through or mediate the older soul/body or mind/matter distinctions. The basic body-building material of the genetic code produced human beings who feel and think in amazingly complex ways. They engage in a wide range of social and cultural activities which build up the human species. The better these activities develop, the more the genes will thrive. There is, then, a constant and necessary interaction between genes and culture. A relatively single or basic unit of culture with its necessary genetic component is called a culturgen.[10] At this stage in his work and in a subsequent more popularized version of this research co-authored again with Lumsden under the title *Promethean Fire* Wilson is at great pains to give proper credit and perspective to social and cultural factors and not to be as reductionist as the early work tended to appear to be.

Perhaps the best presentation of the specifically ethical elements in Wilson's thought is to be found in his recent book called *Biophilia*. This is a text rather uncharacteristic of Wilson in that is is basically a set of personal reminiscences over the number of years in which he has been active as a conservation oriented biologist. But he addresses ethical issues here in quite specific fashion. There are also the quite clear patterns of surface and depth structure now made explicit in terms of some basic methodologies of ethics.

Just as the world of the phenotype tends to be a more biologically set and orderly area, the world of the genotype tends to be the area of biological innovation and new possibilities. Wilson thinks that the world of science is more phenotypical and set while the world of art and imagination is more genotypical and creative. He thinks that we need to be able to integrate the two in a productive synthesis.

In ethical terms this means that we tend to have a surface, scientific ethic which is filled with right-sounding moral strictures, but we need to complement this with the instinctive impulses which we deeply feel bind us to the inner biological rhythms and creative drives of nature. We have to have a sense of belonging and thriving nurtured by our biologically natural origins. This sense is what Wilson terms technically, biophilia.[11] Culture is built up as the deep biological forces that conceived us send inchoate and emotive signals which we can then rationally organize in scientific ways. But the real impetus and strength of any culture is not so much its science but its sense of imagination. Science without this imaginative reverence and respect for the unknown and mysterious will simply pollute its own wells. The crisis in environmental ethics is symptomatic of a wider crisis in our culture. We must be able to tap our hidden resources. This is done more in the world of art, poetry, metaphor and analogy than in the world of hard rational science.[12] This is so because the very mechanisms of genetics work by the overlappings, interplays and meldings of genetic materials which are the deep source of metaphoric, analogous and imaginative interactions. In the reaction and relationship of cultures to their genetic origins, we must again prioritize those origins.

Medicine is an art not a science. It uses the highly organized rational elements of science as much as it can, but when it lets itself become dominated by science then it loses its imaginative heart and soul. It becomes divorced from its inner sense of harmony and continuity with the workings of inner biological rhythms. We have to have a sense of deeply cooperating with nature in order to manipulate it rather than trying so much manipulation of things that we feel no longer deeply a part of the natural processes.

This oscillation between thought and emotion, organization and intuition must also work in the ethical sphere. Just as science has tended too much to dominate our present culture, so we have tried too much to systematize ethics. We have to be aware that ethics is much more an art than a science. A graceful and elegant solution to a complex dilemma is better than a rigidly dogmatic solution. There must be a constant place for ethical growth and revision. This can only take place in a cultural environment of imaginative and creative openness. There must be an inner harmony or teleology in the workings of thought and emotion, conscious and unconscious which is in constant close intuitive contact with the biologically phenotypic and genotypic forces which give and nurture life.

While Wilson is certainly the central figure in the move to a biologically based ethic there are a number of others who should be mentioned. Gunther S. Stent in a still landmark article in one of the early volumes of the then and now trailblazing medical ethics journal, *The Hastings Center Report*, outlined a program for medical ethics which is based securely on a recognition of surface and depth factors in human psychological and biological experience.[13] He begins by pointing out two kinds of scientism. They are hard-core and soft-core scientism. The hard-core scientist is the ultimate rationalist. Stent thinks that this approach fails especially in biological science because there are simply too many observed biological dynamics which will not fit into the patterns of pure scientific logic. But he thinks that soft-core science fails even more in that it is really just a weak and not fully formulated scientific approach which romanticizes the possibilities of science in the solution of not only scientific but ethical problems.

Biology especially is an area where, given the richness of living organisms' growth, development and creativity, a hard and fast scientific pattern of any kind cannot be adopted. Rather we must be eager and able to listen to the deeper signals our inner biology and psychology send to us. This will make us view ethics not so much as a search for pat, certain or ultimate answers, but rather as an exploratory imaginative journey filled with the excitement of ever undiscovered goals.

The fact that Gunther Stent is a rather distinguished professor of molecular biology at the University of California at Berkeley makes his critique of rationalistic scientism even more cogent. He has also followed up this seminal article with a provocative book exploring these themes.[14] Again the fundamental provocative invitation is to empathize with the biopsychosocial rhythms which create and nurture us in our journey into ever further experience and understanding.

The most fundamental question about the nature of these biological rhythms is whether they are merely haphazard or if they have some sort of in-built direction. Is the genetic deck of cards which contains the map of life basically in an unshuffled and disorganized state or is the hand played out according to some rather clear plan of action? The very fact that we talk at all of a genetic map shows that there is some kind of plan or teleology at work. Two other authors have made considerable contributions to our knowledge of the nature of this teleology. Leon Kass in *Toward a More Natural Science: Biology and Human Affairs* takes on the commonly held view that Darwin himself held that there really are no clear directions to natural selection. But Kass notes that such teleological and purposeful terms as useful, important, purpose, adapted, fit, the good of each being, profitable, harmful, beneficial, injurious, advantageous, good, tendency, success, welfare, improvement, low, high, scale of nature and absolute perfection occur on practically every page of *The Origin of Species*. He goes on to group these kinds of usages into references to tendencies, purposes, alterabilities, perfections, directions, adaptations and excellences.[15] There seems to be a movement to betterment in biological affairs, an attempt to perfect the workings of life.

This would also mean that what we have come to call the higher life forms really are higher. It would also maintain that the human form of life is the highest of which we have common experience. Put in more traditional terms, this would mean that the emergence of the human soul brings a new and higher richness to life. It would then be the task of ethics and morality to be most enhancing of this teleological development. The materialist objection would counter that there is no evidence that matter, inert or living, has any capacity to engender or to support the soul. But this rests on a materialist assumption in the first place. Might not the common human experience, documented from the time of the most primitive humanoids, of reaching and searching for the highest spiritual ideals allow at least equally if not more so for a spiritualist assumption. The destiny of matter is spirit or soul and it always moves toward that direction.[16] Even our intimations of immortality should not be discounted and they may be real and genuine clues as to where we are going.[17] Our practice of the virtues would be in harmony with this perfecting teleology so that we can both in metaphor and in truth consider setting our sights very high indeed. The practice of the virtues would find its home environment in an optimstic experience of biopsychosocial perfectioning.

The distinguished evolutionary biologist Ernst Mayr is more cautious about the directions of teleological perfectionism. Rather than looking towards large overarching biological patterns or movements, he is content to note on a smaller scale that there are clearly discernible biological configurations which seem to be somewhat pragmatically self-contained. Within the workings of a larger organism, for instance, there are smaller biological working systems. An example of such a system might be the human endocrinological or digestive system. Within their own limits and on their own terms there is a cooperative working together in the purposive-like activity of contributing to the health of the larger bodily units. Mayr terms this kind of activity teleonomic rather than teleological. [18]

At least in order not to fall into an overly naive optimism in the practice of virtue ethics we might be well advised to work along teleonomic rather than teleological lines. There are more than enough patternings to be discovered and worked within this more modified form. Also a teleonomic approach rings more true to the actual practice of medicine and medical ethics. In this age of medical specializations it really is impossible for one physician to handle all bodily systems, so there is the parcelling out of the work. Once involved in a particular specialty one notes the inner rhythms and harmonies in that area with a view to curing and enhancing their productive possibilities.

Much the same thing happens in ethical work. We take into account the wider picture in which the patterns of ethical life are played out but tend to focus on just what part of the picture is unclear with a view to clarification and reconstruction. The caring for or the curing of the most debilitated teleonomic structure or structures will most likely enhance the growth and development of all the biological, psychological and social structures which form the larger teleological human framework in which we live, move and have our being.

Memorial is a small hospital in McAllen, Texas where patients who "drop in" are often poor Mexican-Americans. Partly because of their poverty, they are often sicker than patients who live further north, in say, Houston. John Smythers, an ethics consultant at University of Texas Medical Branch, was asked one day to go to McAllen to facilitate discussion of a situation involving a Mexican-American farmhand.

Jose Favilla, the 45-year-old farmhand, had been brought into the emergency room at Memorial with a severe concussion, received when he fell off a tractor. His attending, Dr. Smith, is worried that there may have been a considerable insult to Mr. Favilla's brain, and would like to call in a neurosurgeon for a consult, and an operation if necessary.

Unfortunately, Mr. Favilla has no private insurance, no employment insurance, and does not qualify for Medicaid in Texas. The hospital administration is balking at absorbing the cost of a neurosurgeon, which Memorial does not have on staff. But John Sealy Hospital in Galveston, the closest public hospital, is almost 200 miles away, and moving Mr. Favilla is not medically advisable.

Mr. Favilla is married, has three children, and is the sole source of income for his family. He has been unable to find a better job that provides health benefits since unemployment in Texas is higher now than it has been in 17 years.

When Dr. Smythers entered the conference room at Memorial, the administration officer was talking about the financial constraints under which Memorial operated. The chief resident immediately pointed out that the social inequities in that part of Texas were an additional health risk to which nobody should be subjected. Dr. Smythers' appearance provided an excuse to interrupt the discussion. After hearing the details of the case, Dr. Smythers offered his thoughts on the matter:

"It seems to me," he began, "that the discussion is losing its proper focus. I agree there are injustices that affect Mr. Favilla's situation, as well as that of the hospital. But Mr. Favilla needs a surgery consult and perhaps an operation. If he *doesn't* get that specific help, his family will be in worse shape than it was before the accident. Furthermore, there is little we can do directly about the social context. The best we can hope for is that we are acting justly by caring for this one person, and helping to reorder the defective physical system that is preventing him from living the best life he can live under the circumstances."

THE PSYCHOLOGICAL COMPONENT

Just as Charles Darwin was interested in discovering the hidden genotypical founts of human phenotypical biology so he was much concerned with the hidden emotive sources of more clearly rational activity. His book on *The Expression of the Emotions in Man and Animals* is yet to be fully understood and exploited. But Sigmund Freud, at least, knew of the importance of these Darwinian interests. Avid reader as he was of Darwin, it should be no surprise that the two basic psychological drives which he eventually worked out have a strong biological ring to them. So obvious that it took a genius to point it out to us is the fact that at least in our origins all human genetic activity is sexual. Also this genetic sexual activity especially in its phenotypical phases is suffused with some of the strongest possible human emotions. Hence the Freudian libido or sex drive is a highly erotically felt teleonomic thrust in the context of the larger teleology of the total human situation to which it gives rise and continuance.

But Freud came more and more to know that this life-giving sexuality has built into it genetically and emotionally a drive towards its own transformation. All of our genetic material has a certain life span. Our genes are programmed for life and for death. So wrapped up inextricably with the life-giving libido drive is the death drive or thanatos. Freud mapped out the minglings and mergings of these drives in terms of the longings both for life and for death in the twistings and turnings of the Oedipus cycle. Since Freud psychologists and psychiatrists have concentrated at times either on the more unconscious and emotively instinctual elements of his approach or on the more rational and cognitive surface products of the deeper biological and psychological processes.

Erik H. Erikson is certainly one of the most influential of all neo-Freudians.[19] He can be read as stressing the role of irrational drives which must be cognitively overcome at various stages in one's life. He pictures our psychological life as involved in a number of crises in which we must gain some measure of rational control over more diffuse emotional propensities. But each maintaining of control is quite temporary as our emotions again present stage by stage new problems and challenges. Like Freud Erikson situates a number of these key crises in early childhood.

The first crisis is one of basic trust versus basic mistrust. It occurs during early infancy. The second crisis occurs about age four. Here inchoate fears of shame and doubt must be integrated into rational autonomy. At around age five we face a crisis of initiative versus guilt. Between ages six and eleven we must deal with industry versus inferiority. Perhaps the most famous Eriksonian crisis surfaces during adolescence. It is called the identity crisis and has to do with the clarification of personal identity versus identity diffusion. In our early adult life we must reconcile intimacy and isolation, in middle-age generosity versus stagnation, in older life integrity versus despair.

The times of life assigned by Erikson to the various crises have been rather widely moved forward and backward in the actual application of the theories. I suspect that quite a fruitful application of the theory could be made to the stages in the training of a young physician from the infancy days of early medical school until the seemingly settled attainment of a secure and solid practice of medicine. Depending upon what kind of a physician you might be dealing with at a particular stage you almost certainly will be getting a different type of ethical input to your case. Personal physician self-perception influences every ethical decision made sometimes in very dramatic fashion.

Jim Jones is a medical student completing a four week rotation in surgery at Memorial Hospital. Mr. Phillips has been transferred from the medical service, where he has been treated for prostate cancer. He is scheduled to undergo bilateral orchiectomy (castration), and Jim is told by the surgeon to do a lumbar puncture preparatory to spinal anesthesia. Jim has done several lumbar punctures before, but still feels uncertain of himself.

Ever since Mr. Phillips was transferred to surgery, he has been calling Jim "Dr. Jones," and Jim's fellow students, the resident and the head nurse have told him to let that practice continue. As the nurse put it: "The patient will have more confidence in your competence if he believes you are a doctor." But a few hours before the lumbar puncture, the attending mentioned to Mr. Phillips that Jim is a student.

The patient was furious. He had been told that there are serious if unlikely risks associated with lumbar puncture, e.g. bleeding, infection, paralysis, pain, and possibly death. "Do you mean to say that I'm about to be operated on by an incompetent student? I'm a guinea pig?" Mr. Phillips screamed. Jim heard Mr. Phillips complain, and suddenly became uncertain of his own skill. When the attending came out of Mr. Phillips' room, Jim said, "I'm not sure I can do this. Mr. Phillips doesn't have any confidence in me, and I've not performed the procedure very often in the past."

Jim is having a crisis of confidence. Medical students often have to deal with patients who distrust their competence. If you were the attending physician, with a responsibility both to Jim and to Mr. Phillips, how would you respond to Jim's crisis? If you were the medical student, how would you respond to Mr. Phillips' accusation that you were incompetent? Finally, if you were the patient, how would you feel about a procedure being performed on you by a third year medical student?

Mary Johnson, a 66-year-old widow admitted to Memorial

Hospital initially with renal failure, has unexpectedly become a "problem" for the ICU. Shortly after being admited and placed on dialysis, Ms. Johnson had a stroke and has been unable to communicate with anyone for four weeks, when she was intubated. Since then the medical team has been unable to wean her from the ventilator. She is often agitated, exhibits some comprehension, and, generally, seems mentally alert. She has been fitted with a feeding tube, and is receiving IV antibiotics. Ms. Johnson also has a history of heart disease, and has apparently been experiencing angina. She has several times extubated herself, has been reintubated each time, and the attending physician wants to perform a tracheotomy.

Ms. Johnson has lived with her two unmarried sisters for 20 years, and has not been in contact with her two sons for the same length of time. One of her sisters is suffering from basal cell carcinoma of the head and neck, and can play no role in Ms. Johnson's care. The other sister is extremely distraught, and under a great deal of pressure as the sole decisionmaker in the family. She visits Ms. Johnson every day,and seems to think that she understands what she hears even if she can't speak.

Most of the medical team think that Ms. Johnson's multiple systems failure is beginning to overwhelm her. The resident, however, believes that each of her problems can be treated with some significant probability of success. He calls a conference of the medical team, two social workers, Ms. Johnson's sister and Memorial's ethics consultant, Dr. Jones.

Dr. Jones has talked to several members of the team, including the head nurse and resident, and can tell that there is a major disagreement about how aggressive treatment should be. Dr. Jeffries, the attending, is in favor of reducing treatment and not reintubating if Ms. Johnson extubates herself again. The decision, of course, is up to the sister.

At the conference the resident, to Dr. Jones' surprise, was passive. He disagreed with the attending's presentation of the situation only minimally. The presentation very forcefully impressed upon Ms. Johnson's sister the bleakness of the situation if she could not be weaned from the ventilator. We will return to this conference, and the approach the attending took.

The next day the resident decided to take a risk. He wanted to give Ms. Johnson one more chance to breathe on her own, so he turned off the ventilator, and was prepared to reintubate. Ms.

Johnson did start to breathe unassisted, and is now recovering slowly while still receiving dialysis. What is interesting about this case is that the resident displayed a deferential meekness in his public interaction with the attending. Yet he also displayed courage and initiative in those actions he performed outside the surveillance of the attending. This is an example of a resident at a stage in his moral development in which he is striving to define his own identity while still needing some approval from more experienced clinicians.

Mary Johnson's attending physician, Dr. Jeffries, is an experienced physician who has very definite views about life extending technologies. He does not believe they are appropriate for patients who have chronic, terminal illnesses, or who have chronic illnesses with multiple systems breakdowns and are age 65 or older. While he generally respects his patients' autonomy, he will use his powers of persuasion and authority to get a patient or a decision-making surrogate to make the choices *he* thinks are appropriate.

Before the conference previously mentioned, Dr. Jones had arrived at the ICU early in order to determine what were the conflicting views. The resident told him, "I disagree with most of the team" but did not specify how. Hence, it surprised Dr. Jones when the resident expressed his views so timidly at the conference.

Dr. Jeffries arrived at the conference late. He sat down opposite Ms. Johnson's sister, and without wasting time, he ran through the litany of his patient's problems. Near the end of his presentation, he asked Ms. Johnson's sister if she wanted Ms. Johnson reintubated should she extubate herself that night. The woman looked perplexed, asked if that would involve any pain, and when Dr. Jeffries said they would use sufficient sedatives to prevent pain, she quietly said "No – she wouldn't want to live like this."

The conversation was dominated by Dr. Jeffries, although Dr. Jones tried to ensure that the legal process granting Ms. Johnson's sister legal authority was clearly initiated. He also tried to make it clear to her that she had a right to determine the course of treatment. Nonetheless, Dr. Jeffries was completely in charge of the conversation. His manner with Ms. Johnson's sister was direct and kind, but he allowed very little in the way of probing possible alternatives.

Do Dr. Jeffries and the resident fit well in the scheme of development articulated by Erikson? Could the singleness of purpose Dr. Jeffries exhibited degenerate into stagnation?

Stressing very strongly the cognitive approach to ethics is the pioneering work of Lawrence Kohlberg. In his work there is a grounding of ethics securely back on Plato. Two aspects of Plato's thought are most salient. There is a stress on the ultimately rational basis of ethics, but there is also a clear recognition that ethics is radically and basically virtue ethics. In other words Kohlberg is concerned in a contemporary setting to explain how the virtues can be taught and to present a plan for this teaching.

In explaining this platonic point of view Kohlberg is convinced that virtue is basically knowledge of the good. If we really clearly know the good, we will choose to do it. The task of ethics is to make the good ever more clear. This is done by clarifying the principles of ethics. In true platonic form Kohlberg thinks that we already possess in an inchoate way these principles. The task of the ethician is to draw these out of us so that we can ever better understand them. The teaching of ethics is done by a socratic question and answer method rather than by a dogmatic statement of principles. This methodology introduces a rather strong pragmatism. Only in the working out of questions and answers in actual practice can the higher levels of self-knowledge and virtue be developed.

Clearly this approach is congenial to a great deal of medical practice. In the clinical situation so much is learned by question and answer. A good supervising clinician must rely on the expertise of residents and even of medical students in the attempt to solve complex and recalcitrant medical problems. The question and answering which go on in the clinical situation are anything but theoretical. The conclusions reached are immediately brought into play. While thought and action here are almost synonymous there does remain a premium on intellectual expertise. The more you know the more you can act well. But your actions are then subject to cognitive review by yourself and by other members of the health care team. One also has the sense that there is a calling up of these principles for action out of the depths of knowledge and experience. This is most especially true for ethical principles. Understood in this way physicians have more than something of a case when they say that they already know ethics and do not need a professional ethicist to instruct them. This is true if we are talking of the ethicist coming into a clinical situation and presenting a lecture on ethics as a contribution to the solution of a case. But if the ethicist acts as a facilitating member of the team just as all the other team members do, then there is the possibility of virtuous education and learning by all members of the team including the ethicist.

Kohlberg thinks that an individual tends to operate at one or another ethical level or stage. There is more or less a single ethical principle which is employed at any given stage. It will be the job of the ethicist and other members of the team to bring to light just what principles may be involved and to suggest a possible move to a higher level of ethical judgment and action. Like Erikson, Kohlberg assigns some rather ideal ages at which the various stages of moral development occur but these might be malleable for different people in different situations. Because he considers justice to be the highest virtue, all development in morality involves an ever greater awareness and sensitivity to the demands and needs of others. There are basically six stages of moral development. The stages are grouped into three levels. There is a basic set of underlying reasons at each stage for the drafting and employment of moral rules of action.

At the first more primitive level of moral development moral values reside in external physical happenings and needs rather than in relations between people. The rights and duties of others are not totally excluded here but the stress is on the fulfillment of personal needs and desires in terms of a good deal of self-gratification in rather materialistic ways. The first stage of ethical action at this level is one in which the main moral concerns have to do with obedience and punishment. There is a deference to superior power or prestige and a desire to avoid making any unnecessary trouble. Responsibility is as much as possible put onto the shoulders of others. While Kohlberg assigns this stage to around age ten, this sort of situation regularly occurs with the young medical student or even resident who often, in order to protect personal home turf, knuckles under to authority.

At the University of Texas Medical Branch, third year medical students are required to attend a five week internal medicine ethics clerkship. Each session is directed by a member of the Institute for the Medical Humanities and a clinician. At a recent session, Dennis, a student, wanted to talk about a situation that troubled him.

Dennis: A 68-year-old woman with late stage liver cancer was admitted for the third time last week, and it was unlikely she would survive this admission. She was coherent, but in a great deal of pain. Of course, she wanted pain medication. Her first

147

night she was screaming and the intern ordered tylenol with codeine, which we both knew would not help her very much. I asked the intern whether we shouldn't give her enough morphine to kill the pain, but he refused to do so.

Dr. Kluge (the clinician): Why did he not order the morphine?

Dennis: When I asked him, he said the resident on call told him not to. He didn't want to contravene the resident's decision.

Dr. Kluge: But it's standard care to provide morphine in a situation like that. Assuming the intern was just following orders, why didn't the resident want to follow procedure?

Dennis: She apparently thought a dose of morphine sufficient to alleviate the pain might kill the patient. She didn't want to make that decision on her own.

Dr. Jones (the ethicist): But why would she not discuss this with the attending taking care of the patient? We might understand her unwillingness to harm the patient on her own initiative, but the patient shouldn't be allowed to suffer a great deal.

Dennis: It was 2 a.m. According to the intern, the resident would have to have awakened the attending, and she didn't want to do that.

Dr. Kluge: Why not?

Dennis: She was afraid to.

Dr. Kluge: Well, first of all, if we are hearing the whole story, she had the authority to order the morphine. Secondly, if she didn't want to make a risky decision on her own, she should have called the attending. We expect our residents to do that, if they need to. Thirdly, the intern could have called the attending.

Dennis: But he was afraid to contravene the authority of the resident.

Dr. Jones: What finally happened?

Dennis: I spent almost the whole night with the patient, holding her hand and talking her through the pain as best I could.

Dr. Kluge: And the next day?

Dennis: The attending was very angry at not being informed of the problem, and ordered the morphine.

At around age 13 Kohlberg thinks that there is more of an awareness of the needs and rights of other people. Still at this stage within level one the catering to the needs of others is to insure one's own desires and securities. There is nonetheless an early awareness of the reciprocity of rights and duties and so there is a move to some type of egalitarianism.

At the second level there is a development of the recognition of social interaction in a stress of maintaining conventional patterns of order. A good deal of emphasis is placed on the types of roles that are to be played out in interpersonal relationships. These roles are much influenced by the fulfilling of the expectations of others.

The first stage of this level, which Kohlberg places at about age 15, involves a good deal of stereotypical behavior with the expectation that one will be perceived as basically a good person. There is the need to conform to the majority in thought and behavior.

The second stage of this level recognizes the real values of authority and social order on their own grounds and not so much for the sake of personal security. Here an often strong sense of duty mandates a respect for authority and social structures. While age 19 is assigned to this stage, the medical student or resident may see very neat strengths in the structures and hierarchies of medical practice and very much value them for their own sakes.

There is a distinction that can be drawn between "authority" and "authoritarian". One can be an authority without being authoritarian, and vice versa. An authority wields *legitimate* power, while an authoritarian does not. What counts as *legitimate* power may vary across societies, but it is generally recognized by members of a society in paradigmatic cases.

Residents often make the distinction, even if they are not always aware of it, in their responses to attending physicians. Consider the following situation, which involves the use of electroconvulsive shock therapy (ECT) for severe manic-depressive illness that is not responsive to drug treatment.

Roger Smith, a 55-year-old man has attempted suicide several times. He was admitted each time and prescribed several different anti-depressants to treat endogamous depression. He had, until his first suicide attempt, been apparently stable, held down a job for 20 years, and raised a family with whom he has good relationships. But he had been morose for six months before the first attempt at suicide and his wife and children had grown very worried.

After the third admission, the attending psychiatrist, Dr. Williams, and the resident, Dr. Coover, agreed that he was unresponsive to drug therapy and had had some troubling side effects from one of them. Tofranil had caused rapid heartbeat, nausea, and diarrhea and a severe skin rash.

Despite the public concern about ECT, it has succeeded in several recent randomized clinical trials in reducing depressive symptoms, and is often considered the treatment of choice when a patient is suicidal, unresponsive to drug therapy and develops severe side effects to anti-depressants. Drs. Williams and Coover had the following conversation one afternoon:

Dr. Williams: I'd like to try ECT, but Mr. Smith is terribly frightened by it.
Dr. Coover: So am I and I know from talking to him that Mr. Smith won't agree to it. From what I know about ECT, the risks outweigh the benefits. The memory loss can be severe, and, frankly, it *looks* frightening. I've seen it done.

Dr Williams explained the results of the recent clinical trials and pointed out that it is not painful, the amnesia is either temporary or mild and the frequency of death is well below 1 per cent. Dr. Coover remained unconvinced.

Dr. Coover: Look – Mr. Smith will refuse. We have three choices: 1) we can have him declared incompetent; 2) we can pressure him to agree to ECT; 3) we can just continue the discussion of risks and benefits with him. I'll refuse to participate in this decision if you don't let Mr. Smith make the decision.
Dr Williams: Mr. Smith will very likely either kill himself and harm his family if we don't use ECT. Let me tell you a story.

Dr. Williams then told Dr. Coover of a similar situation that occurred to a psychiatric resident who had persuaded his attending not to use ECT. The patient had gone on a killing spree and, while the resident never felt completely comfortable using ECT, and was a strong proponent of anti-depressant drugs as they were developed over the years, he accepted the use of ECT as a last line of defense. At the end of the story, Dr. Williams said: "I was that resident."

Dr. Coover finally relented to this extent. He insisted that they try to persuade Mr. Smith with the least possible amount of coercion. Combining coercion with ECT intensifies the fear reluctant patients have about the effects of ECT. But Dr. Coover was convinced by the experience of Dr. Williams, and recognized his humane concern for the patient and his family. In the end, Dr.

Williams did have to threaten Mr. Smith with involuntary commitment to persuade him to agree to ECT. Dr. Coover was never comfortable with that decision. But he did acknowledge the role of authority in enabling health care practitioners to make hard choices without completely undermining the self-respect of patients. Perhaps the most important question for you to pose about the legitimacy of authority is this: Is the authority willing to provide *good reasons* for a decision, or does he or she simply rely on the power of his or her *office* to support the decision?

The third level is an altruistic one in which the individual recognizes that there are moral standards which can only be upheld if there is individual and group cooperation. At this level rights and duties are more objectified and codified.

The first stage of this level involves a contractual legalistic orientation. Duty is, however, still defined somewhat negatively as the avoidance of violating the rights of others. This kind of ethical awareness might develop at about age 25. The present climate of fear of malpractice litigation might well place many a physician of whatever age into this sort of a moral configuration.

Most physicians will acknowledge that they have a duty to tell patients the truth about their condition, on the basis of the principle that everyone has a right to equal respect. The duty to respect persons is useful, in that it can result in cooperation among patients, families and physicians, and cooperation is an important element of good medicine. Indeed, cooperation can transform merely technically correct medicine into *healing*.

But truth-telling can also be an element in malpractice suits. If a patient is not told the truth, she or her family may sue the physician for malpractice if something goes wrong. Hence, some physicians can "tell the truth" mechanically, to avoid legal disputes.

An excellent example of the harm of such a mechanical approach to the duty of truth-telling occurs in the movie (and novel) *Dad*. One of the protagonists of the story is an elderly man whose wife has just suffered (but survived) a serious myocardial infarction. His family has gathered around him and the setting becomes an opportunity for the old man and his son (a yuppie stockbroker) to re-establish ties of affection and respect. The setting also becomes an opportunity for the son to establish similar ties to *his* son, a rebellious teenager.

This is the context in which the old man is discovered to have cancer. The "C-word" carries a heavy meaning for him, of which

151

only his son is aware. The son begs the doctor not to tell his father that he has cancer:

> "You don't know what that word means to him. Please, please don't tell him. Let me tell him – I know how to do it."

Sometime during the next few days the old man descends into a dark coma from which he almost doesn't return. The son discovers that the doctor has told the father that he has cancer, under the guise that the patient has a right to know. The sub-text of this part of the story is that the physician is so afraid of a malpractice suit that he loses sight of the fears and needs of his patient, ironically committing malpractice in the process.

Notice that the son did not ask the physician to lie. He only wanted to ensure that someone sensitive to the old man's terror be the one to tell him of his condition.

Respecting the rights of patients by telling them the truth is indeed an important "negative virtue," if we are interested in protecting patients from coercion. But the moral of *Dad* is that we often have to let the positive virtue of *love* shape the way we express our respect to patients as persons. In other words, duty does not exhaust the repertoire of moral concepts we need to preserve humane relationships in health care. Truly to respect persons is to be responsive to their needs and fears, not merely to follow legal or ethical *rules*.

This level's second stage recognizes that moral principles are true and correct because of an inner logic. Such rules are universal in their application. Kohlberg thinks that a person at or over age 30 might be able to have a conscience well-formed by this kind of ethical universalism.

At times Kohlberg has suggested that there might be a possible seventh stage beyond the six basic ethical stages which he has been most concerned to discuss and develop. At this stage moral values would reside in the basic relation of self to all of reality. Moral action at this stage would be in the context of a non-egoistic experience of the larger rhythms and realities of life and death of which an individual is only rather a small part. This would be a mystical, religious experience of a fundamental ground of hope in the face of despair and death. Given the kind of dealing with life and death which is a daily aspect of the practice of medicine, there are ample occasions for both physician and patient to experience and put into practice this stage.[20]

THE SOCIAL SECTOR

With the rise of classical forms of deontology and utilitarianism a good deal of virtue ethics suffered an eclipse. Any revival of virtue ethics in the contemporary setting will have to take into account the important developments in both of these approaches. But they might well be incorporated into the larger frame of virtue ethics. One way of doing this is to consider them as homologous to the already discussed biological and psychological elements in the biopsychosocial structure which forms the essential frame for virtue ethics.

In this way act deontology which concentrates on the particular ethical feeling, sometimes called conscience, of acting rightly or wrongly, would be akin to the emotive aspects of the psychological part of the ethical frame. Act utilitarianism would also be seen as an emotive ethic. Rather than concentrating on a particular duty-filled ethical feeling as in act deontology, there would here be a concentration on the maximization of pleasure and minimization of pain, the sort of pursuit of happiness ethic enshrined in the American Declaration of Independence.

But deontological thinkers such as Immanuel Kant and W. D. Ross were concerned to think through in a very orderly way the ways in which we ought to organize and understand the more primal ethical emotive drives of act deontology. Kant formulated in what is now often termed rule deontology four versions of what he called the Categorical Imperative. By this he meant that as we think about our feeling of duty or conscience we see that we have certain fundamental absolute duties to each which must be carried out if we are to satisfy the felt need to be ethical. One of these formulations is especially applicable to the field of clinical medical ethics. Kant maintains that we should always treat humanity whether in our own person or in that of another always as an end and never as a means to an end only.

Patients are in a unique position to be exploited and treated as ends for our own purposes. We use them as examples for teaching or subjects for research. Kant wants to make us aware always that each patient and each colleague have an absolute dignity in and of themselves so we must always do our best not to manipulate them.

Another contribution to the thinking through of duty ethics is in the work of W. D. Ross. As noted in the introductory chapter he is often cited as having prioritized three prime duties, autonomy, beneficence and justice. Actually he worked out duties of fidelity, reparation, gratitude, justice, beneficence, self-improvement and non-maleficence. All of these duties were to make sure again of the dignity of each individual person and the need to absolutely respect that dignity. They can omnipresently be applied in medical practice.

When Jeremy Bentham in the 1800s proposed his version of pleasure oriented act utilitarianism he was accused of having devised an ethics for pigs. Responsive to this criticism Bentham worked out the most common form of rule utilitarianism which is an attempt to think through just how we might all best be able to maximize our pleasure and minimize our pain. He called this the Principle of Utility or the Hedonic Calculus. It basically maintains that if the greatest number of people are happy then the chances are best that any single individual will be happy. The principle has wide application in many rather broad social areas but perhaps less specific application in clinical medical ethics where the degree of pleasure possible is already considerably lessened by the disease or injury situation itself. But there may be a good deal of direct application of this principle to the problems of medical staff interpersonal relationships.

Another rule oriented approach to ethics is social contract ethical theory. Some ethicians want to make this a part of deontological ethics in that the contract spells out the duties which we have to each other as a result of that contract. It might also or better be conceived of as part of a utilitarian approach to ethics in that a good social contract would insure as much as possible the greatest happiness of the greatest number with the contract providing the best climate for this outcome. It is important to note that here we are talking about contract in the most basic and general sense. This is not a legal contract but rather a basic understanding of the relationship which we have with other people. This relationship is a more or less understood presupposition of our common working together and our common satisfaction.

One type of such a social contract might be the kind proposed classically by Jean-Jacques Rousseau in the 1700s. This would maintain that we basically trust and respect each other and so can go about the business of interpersonal interactions in a wholesome and constructive way. In the 1600s Thomas Hobbes had proposed quite a different kind of social contract, one based on fear and mistrust. Medical practice often oscillates between these two contractual points of view. A trusting and open physician-patient relationship, often of quite long standing, can suddenly and dramatically change into one of doubt and mistrust. This can often be for the simplest of reasons such as physician impatience or brusqueness. From such sudden turns comes many a malpractice suit.

One of the strongest contemporary ethical theories is the social contract devised by John Rawls in his contemporary classic *A Theory of Justice*. He claims that his theory is a deontological one because it strongly stresses the principles of the social contract rather than their utilitarian consequences.[21] But if the two more classic forms of social contract theory can be seen as utilitarian in trying to build up the greatest happiness for the greatest number, a case can well be made for placing the Rawlsian enterprise in this category.

Four parts of this version of the social contract are of most importance to us. Rawls asks that we think of people as being in a rather imaginary original situation or position. In this situation all people would be as much as possible totally equal with no one having an advantage over another. In the actual real world we have to make our decisions and choices looking through a veil of ignorance in which we can see some possible consequences rather clearly but others not so well. We strive nonetheless to as much as possible make ethical choices which will satisfy the ideal of trying to make the human condition as just a one as possible, to approximate as much as possible the original position. In making these choices two principles play a key role. We should strive as much as possible to secure equal liberty for all parties. In order to do this any strongly committed democratic society must look to the needs of its least advantaged members, for if we do not take care of them they will remain a burden and society will always be the poorer.[22] Rawls' principles are seen by such creative medical ethicists as Norman Daniels to have far-reaching application in questions of distribution of funds for health care.[23]

But no one approach, biological, psychological or social, can answer the needs of clinical medical ethics. There are times when one or the other aspects might be prioritized and other considerations might be of less importance. There is a need to be able to ethically diagnose and prognose well. At times more genotypical or medical aspects of the case demand more attention. At other times surgical or physiological intervention of some sort is more appropriate. In the psychological area there is sometimes need for cool rational argumentation, at other times for more intuitive emotional response. Sometimes our response to the social factors in a medical case should be more instinctive act deontology or utilitarianism; at other times a more complex thinking through of the possibilities of rule deontology or utilitarianism is more appropriate. Most needed is the ability to see all of these parts and pieces of the biopsychosocial frame as forming a larger ethical organic structure where no element or factor is ever ruled out but where each can offer a tool in practice for action in the complexities of the ethical problematic. The habitual ability to use these tools in the most appropriate and effective way is the pragmatic practice known as virtue ethics. What is now most needed in virtue ethics is a study of the techniques for integrating and applying the richness of ethical tools at our disposal.

THE VIRTUE SYNTHESIS

Working out of the tradition established by Thomas Aquinas with the prioritizing of the practical reasoning found in habitually prudential choices, John Finnis in his *Natural Law and Natural Rights* recommends that in ethical decision making we have as much as possible a consistent and harmonious set of purposes and orientations. There should be a kind of wholeness or integrity to our actions. In order to achieve this we should not arbitrarily discount or exaggerate basic ethical values. An aid to this might be the pragmatic attempt to universalize or at least put into a larger context our particular ethical preferences and choices. This will require a certain detachment from the pressures and complexities of the actual situation. We also have to establish a certain consistency in our choices and decisions which might be aided by a rather constant sense of fidelity to our commitments. In this context it would be important not to choose against any basic ethical value. We should choose efficient means to bring about precise and proper ends. While we must act in accord with our personal conscience, we must as much as possible further and foster the social good of the community.[24]

The Institute for the Medical Humanities at the University of Texas has a Ph.D. program in medical humanities. One required course is the clinical ethics practicum, in which Ph.D. candidates participate with an experienced ethics consultant in ethics conferences, bedside consultation and classroom discussion.

Dale is a Ph.D. candidate who is taking the practicum. She worked for several years as a respiratory therapist, studied philosophy as an undergraduate and has become interested recently in the importance of understanding the patients' narratives in framing clinical decisions.

One case in which Dale was involved concerned a 17-year-old son of a working-class family with three other children. George had been admited to John Sealy Hospital after three days of nausea, vomiting and persistent abdominal pain. After a series of GI X-rays and a gastroscopy, George was found to have an obstruction of the small intestine. During exploratory surgery, the surgeon discovered a large pancreatic tumor which had metastasized to the intestine, regional lymph nodes, liver and one kidney. George had undergone two regimens of chemotherapy, and the cancer was still spreading. Surgery was at this point out of the question.

The mother wants to continue chemotherapy, even though the oncologist has told her he believes it will not do any good. George has said that he can't stand continuing to live with the pain and the suffering he is causing his family.

The health care team is inclined to discuss with George the likelihood that he will die within a few months, but his mother is extremely angry that the physicians would do such a thing before trying another series of chemotherapy treatments. They do not want to discuss the situation further with George's family, because of what they perceive as his mother's irrational anger. The patient's right to choose, they say, is absolute anyway, so why engage in a futile discussion with overwrought parents?

Dale, at a conference at which George was discussed by the health care team, was concerned about their attitude. She pointed out that she, and not they, had established a relationship not just with George's mother, but also with his older sister, father and aunt. Dale had indeed had long conversations with George and his family over the last couple of days. She pointed out that there was a great deal about George and his family that they did not know, among which was the fact that George's family were not of one mind about what role George ought to play in the decision-making process. Dale argued:

"How can you make a decision without knowing all the people involved? You owe respect to the patient's family, and in order to discharge that debt you need to discuss the situation with all of them. Maybe you will be able to achieve consensus without violating anyone's rights, while at the same time provide support for a suffering family."

How is Dale responding to an over-emphasis on one value (respect for patient's rights)? Is she right for trying to direct the physicians' focus away from the patient alone? Is she in a special position to balance moral goods, relative to the physicians?

Another classic formulation of the structure of the habitual practice of virtue is provided by Alasdair MacIntyre in the book which more or less instigated the current revival of interest in virtue ethics, *After Virtue*. In order to be involved in the habitual and productive practice of virtue ethics MacIntyre says that we must sense ourselves as belonging to a coherent and complex form of human activity. While he is pessimistic about the possibilities in modern society of providing the coherent framework necessary to a virtue ethic, we might very much see in medical practice just such a frame. The more we can experience ourselves as part of a coherent attempt to solve common problems the better chance we have at setting the proper ethical priorities and making the most efficient ethical choices.

If we are working as constructive members of a team we will be looking to build up the aims and ends of that activity for their own sakes. MacIntyre calls these goods internal to that activity. In medical terms, the purpose and aim of all members of the health care team to bring about care or cure are the basic reasons why we are all involved in the activity. There are external reasons for doing this kind of work as well such as monetary recompense but these reasons must remain secondary or they will deter us and cloud our clinical and ethical judgment. The doctor, nurse or clinical ethician who is primarily concerned about how much money is to be made or how much personal prestige to be built up will not be a very effective practitioner. As a key to help understand the diffrence between goals and aims internal and external to a practice, we might note that the pursuit of internal goods benefits all the people involved in the endeavor, patients and staff alike while the direct pursuit of an external good will usually benefit only one person.

Dr. James is a teaching attending at Memorial Hospital, and has a lucrative private practice. Because of his rigorous schedule, he is often overworked and exhausted. Recently he has started resenting the demands his patients at Memorial, most of them poor, make on him. Often the thought has crossed his mind, "Those patients are getting good, free health care, and they don't even appreciate it."

One day he had a particularly heavy load of private patients in his Gold Coast office and was on call at Memorial. He usually tried to avoid being on call while seeing private patients, but this day followed a holiday, and he had no choice but leave himself open to a scheduling conflict if he wanted to keep his private patients happy.

While examining a woman with gall stones, but who was only there for a six-month checkup, he heard his beeper. He called Memorial and was told the emergency room was extremely crowded with post-holiday accident victims. Angrily he muttered to himself, "Those people at Memorial probably had too much to drink or smoked too much dope last night, and now they want me to patch them up after their irresponsible behavior got them into trouble." He told the ER nurse that he had his own patients to see, but would be over as soon as possible.

All the patients Dr. James had scheduled that morning were there for routine examinations and could have been rescheduled. But rather than risking their ire, and the fees they were prepared to pay him, he spent the whole morning at this office. When he arrived at the ER he saw that all hell had broken loose.

The triage nurse had fallen behind, through no fault of her own, and no other attending had been called since they expected Dr. James to arrive "as soon as possible." One accident victim had been misdiagnosed by an overworked resident, and had died from massive brain hemorrhage. He had, incorrectly, been placed low on the list of priorities. Several other patients had required immediate attention and no one had had time to see them.

Are Dr. James' priorities correctly ordered if the proper aim of medicine is health? Assigning blame for the death or illness of a person is usually neither possible nor appropriate, but has Dr. James' concern for his private patients overwhelmed his sense of responsibility to his patients at Memorial? How would you arrange your priorities if you were motivated both by your calling as a physician and by the temptations of a for-profit health care system?

The pursuit of virtue involves always trying to achieve ever higher standards of excellence. In order to do this we must always be practicing and increasing our technical skills. This advice applies so clearly to the practice of medicine that it needs no further comment.

Because of the need for constant improvement the goals of medical practice are not rigidly fixed, but rather are integral to the profession itself. As medical science and technology advance our goals change and become more optimistic. As we discover new explanations for previous problems and devise new ways of attacking situations our explanations themselves contain a not so hidden evaluation of our previous and present progress. We consider old and outmoded techniques and goals bad, new and improved ones better. Anyone using outmoded techniques is in some sense bad, the people more on the cutting edge are good. So there are ethically evaluative elements embedded in the development of the practice of medicine.

Finally MacIntyre points out that in the practice and pursuit of virtue we need to have a basic internal pleasure, enjoyment and sense of satisfaction in what we are doing. The very deeply dedicated ethical determination to be loyal and constant in the practice of virtue itself can be both a part of this satisfaction and a vital contribution to the attainment of goals and purposes.[25]

As regards the specific use of the ethical options available in the practice of virtue ethics, Ruth Purtilo, who is director of the program in ethics at the Massachusetts General Hospital Institute of Health Professions, outlines a number of points which an ethicist should be most careful about in entering and working in the clinical medical situation.

First, it is important to make sure that the invitation is really to a medical ethicist for a consulting role on the team. It may turn out that what is really being looked for is legal counsel or religious support. The clinical ethicist should not try to play another role. Second, when you do become engaged in the discussion make sure that you have a great deal of respect for the other members of the team, for the patient, the patient's family and anyone else who may be involved. Most consult situations are ones of such emotional tension and strain that total respect for the fragile members of the group is absolutely essential.

Third, listen as though your patient's life depended on it. Often the patient's life does depend on what you are going to say. Recall that often you are called on the case somewhat late in the game when many or all other options or recourse have failed. Do not forget that what you say and do may much affect the lives not only of the patient's family and friends but also the members of the health care team such as nursing or social work staff who may be already in a threatened situation because of the politics of medical power at work in the case.

Fourth, speak as though your own life depended on it. In varying degrees this may be quite true either of your professional life itself or of your ability to function well in the future with the team. Fifth, do not overstay your welcome. There are many cases when just a few well placed remarks are all that are needed in the case. Also because of the fact of being called in late on the scene and because of the almost at times desperate turning to the ethicist for support and help there is a tendency and temptation to take center stage in the discussion. Those who have already been playing the game long and hard will be much put off by this. At any rate the chances of the consulting ethicist being really attuned to the nuances and complexities of a long drawn out case are slim indeed. Be clear; be brief; be gone.

Sixth, as you go leave the opportunity open for follow-up. It is a good technique for teaching to end a class on an uncertain note so as to keep the students interested and tantalized. While a consult should not leave undone what should be commented upon as fully as possible, it is the very nature of an ethical dilemma that there will remain details and loose ends which cannot be completely handled. There may even be a number of other options which it would be quite ethical to take. As a result it is much better to leave with a sense of openness to further change and development than to convey the impression that you have neatly once and for all solved the case.

Seventh, after a particularly tough case or a tiredly long day, take the long way home. Allow yourself leisure time to disengage from the pressure of a case. This will not only provide you with psychological distance you need but will build up a personal attitude of professional distance. You will be able to approach future cases not overburdened by the weight of past or pending cases. And allow yourself the credit of a job well done.[26]

This kind of practical sharing of experience and advice as to how to conduct the project of clinical medical ethics consulting well is vital to the success and progress of those working in such a new, tentative and tense profession. There is now an American-Canadian Society for Bioethics Consultation. Besides having regular workshop meetings, it publishes a newsletter. But a few years before this organization was set up a key conference on clinical medical ethics was held at the University of Tennessee where one of the first and most successful graduate programs in clinical health care ethics was developed. At the end of the meeting the 175 health care professionals involved in the discussions were asked what kind of ethical approach they actually found themselves practicing in clinical work. The majority claimed that they were adherents of an approach to ethics which has long been under a cloud and seldom invoked. They claimed that they were casuists.

Just what is a casuist? It really comes from the Latin word, *casus*, meaning a case. So a casuist is a person who engages in a case study approach to solving ethical problems. For a variety of reasons this appealed to the clinical medical ethicists. Obviously our work is for the most part with individual cases so there is very much the building up of ethical expertise from the experience of a number of complex cases. Clinical medical ethics is also regularly taught using a case study approach and there are many collections of medical ethics cases now in print to cater to this need. But there was a dominant school of casuistical writers who flourished from the sixteenth to the eighteenth century. These were regularly religious clerics who were concerned with proper sacramental practice in their churches, but in the course of this they developed a most highly nuanced pragmatic methodology for dealing with the ethical complexities of case study.

One of the major papers at the Tennessee conference was an exposition by Albert R. Jonsen of the methodology of casuistry. A number of the basic factors at play in casuistry were rather clearly mapped out. A collection of cases in a typical casuistic manual of this period would contain a very large number of paradigm cases. They might be grouped under one or more general headings such as the Ten Commandments or the Seven Deadly Sins. In dealing with these cases it is most important to see how one case is like but yet quite unlike another case, so there is a strong stress on the role of analogy in ethical reasoning. Circumstances of each case will much dictate this likeness and unlikeness. There is a minute attention to detail, especially in the nuances of personal intention and preference in each case. A working carefully through a number of cases ought to produce a certain number of working principles or maxims. Then we have to determine just how strong or arguable these maxims are. One principle or maxim may be in real or seeming conflict with another, so we have to seek some method of resolving the problems.[27]

In their recent study, *The Abuse of Casuistry*, which is not only a history of casuistry but a proposal for a carefully crafted contemporary version of pragmatic importance and significance, Jonsen and Toulmin begin by mapping out some of the older Aristotelian tradition differences between theoretical and practical knowledge.[28] Theoretical knowledge is idealized. It deals with abstractions which can be thought of and discussed with near absolute precision. Practical knowledge is concrete. Our working in this area is imprecise and rests in some measure on direct experience of the actual complexities of things. Theoretical knowledge is always and ever true and so is atemporal, while practical knowledge of particular cases may very well change and develop over a period of time. Theoretical arguments are necessary. They must fit into the pattern of scientific or logical explanation where they rigidly find their home. Practical argumentation is presumptive in that we always have to be alert to the exception in a situation which may point us to greater knowledge in another presumptive case.

A theoretical argument would begin with a major premise which would take a rather abstract or universal position. An example would be a theorem of geometry or a law of physics. A minor premise would detail the specifics of a particular case so that the major principle could then be applied in the case.

A practical argument would rather reach a kind of general principle or maxim or warrant based on the details of particular facts and situations. Any conclusion reached would be provisional and temporary. There would always be an alertness for counter-arguments which would arise as new facts and circumstances would call for a re-assessment of the situation. This kind of argumentation is classically seen in the ever changing profiles of standard medical practice. A clinical rule is at the very strongest only a warrant for acting as best we can in the situation at this point. The wisdom of accumulated medical practice dictates constant revision of these warrants as new techniques and the experience of their use develop.[29]

In a key lecture at a recent meeting of the Society for Bioethics Consulation Albert Jonsen mapped out in considerable detail the precise mechanisms employed by the classical casuists in the working through of the various facets of practical reasoning.[30] The methodology is highly rhetorical in style in that it works with what would be reasonably persuasive arguments in the building up of a case. In this law and medicine for all their deep differences would share with applied ethics a common approach. While casuistry reinstates the role of persuasive argumentation to the ethical forum, it also wants to make sure that this argumentation is also reasonable. So it concentrates on making sure that any ethical warrant or maxim such as "tell the truth" or "respect the dignity of another person" is made relevant in terms of the details pertaining to particular persons, places, times and actions. Four key components of the casuistic scheme clarify the reasonableness of persuasive rhetoric.

First, a number of cases are grouped in a taxonomy. This is just what has been done for some time in the development of medical ethics. We have a number of topics and cases which are grouped along the same lines in almost all medical ethics texts and anthologies. There are cases about death and dying, about abortion, about genetics and genetic engineering, about artificial insemination and surrogate parenting, about informed consent and confidentiality, about truth-telling and patient rights, about public policy as regards the distribution of health care funds, about research and experimentation. While the cases within a certain grouping are very analogous to each other, there are certain paradigm cases which govern the parameters of the debate. Cases such as Quinlan, Saikewicz and Conroy dominate the death and dying debate. Roe versus Wade dominates all debate in the abortion issue. The matter of Mary Beth Whitehead is the surrogate parenting issue. The Tarasoff case is the central paradigm in questions of confidentiality; Canterbury versus Spence and ZeBarth in informed consent.

These paradigm cases often are centered on a certain maxim such as in the Quinlan case that parents should make the kind of termination of life decisions a now incompetent person would make if that person knew this to be a terminal situation. But the maxims used in these paradigm cases must be tested by trying out their application in other analogous cases. A very strong maxim might well stand up to this test and so remain applicable across quite a number of cases. As the details and circumstances of the cases change these maxims would come under more and more attack until the pressure builds to switch to another paradigm with another maxim operative. Even when a maxim is functioning very strongly in a series of cases there will always be counter-arguments so that we should never think of a maxim as being so ironclad as to override any contrary considerations. At best a maxim can only be pragmatically applied.

Second, morphology proposes a format for the structure of argumentation which might lead us from one paradigm to another. General morphology notes that there are certain features which characterize all moral action. There is, for instance, a certain causality operative in all moral situations. Often dramatic consequences can be traced to the decisions and actions which brought them about. This tracing can be more clearly done in moral matters because the role of intent and execution is much more evident. Individuals or groups must take responsibility for intentions and actions as well. Often omission to do something when the possibility for action is open can be construed as morally the same as taking overt action. Attention must be paid to what are the directly intended consequences of an intended act as distinct from unavoidable secondary results.

Special morphology notes that there are moral activities which are more proper to specified fields of particularly moral activity. In the field of medical ethics this would refer to the need to work with highly precise medical indications. There would also be a need to consult and incorporate patient preferences. The role of the family as well as other members of the health care team would be crucial. Considerations of quality of life might be critical. The biases and preferences of physicians have to be carefully noted. The psychological state of physician, patient, patient's family and other members of the health care team much influences decisions made. Socioeconomic factors more and more influence and even dictate crucial decisions.

A technique is used in morphology called parsing the case. The term comes from the field of grammar and rhetoric. Here the consideration of the tense of a verb, the case of a noun, the function of a word in a sentence as subject, object, adjective, adverb or proposition helps to explicate the inner workings of language. In much the same way we can take apart the structure of a moral argument rather as we can take apart the structure of a sentence. The larger sentence structure might be considered to be a theorem or theory. This would be a rather general ethical norm such as the one forbidding murder. A moral maxim would be fitted to this general theory but only because we see the maxim at work in a number of analogous cases, not because we deductively apply the theorem and so over-impose it on the case. The grounds for the use of the maxim must be checked in terms of the precise circumstances of the individual cases. A stronger or weaker claim can then be made for using the maxim and its connection with the warrant theorem will then also be stronger or weaker. Place must always be made for rebuttals and exceptions as no maxim with its overriding theorem will ever perfectly fit an actual case or set of cases.

It's easy enough these days to say of an adult, competent, terminally ill patient that she has a right to choose the course of her treatment. But the cognitively impaired elderly in very poor health pose complications which can only be evaluated by using analogy. Consider the following case:

Henry is an 82-year-old man who was admitted to Memorial Hospital's ER because he was breathing with difficulty. He was dehydrated, malnourished, anemic and had a urinary tract infection. His primary diagnosis, however, was pneumonia – once known as "the old man's friend."

Henry was treated with antibiotics, packed red blood cells, a Foley catheter, and IV fluids, electrolytes and vitamins. He had to be fed though a nasogastric tube. He was conscious, but had a very low level of cognitive capacity as far as anyone could tell. His eldest daughter and son came to visit him, the daughter as often as her own family and work responsibilities would permit, and the son nearly every day.

After a week of hospitalization with virtually no communication with anyone, Henry was judged to have senile dementia. The prognosis for senile dementia is progressive brain degeneration and eventual death. It was unlikely that Henry would live, even in the best of circumstances, longer than five years; and he would almost certainly be completely dependent.

None of Henry's children were capable either of caring for him themselves or of paying for home care, so it would be unlikely that he would be able to live anywhere except in a state run nursing facility. It was likely that Henry's pneumonia could be treated successfully with antibiotics, but his life down the road looked grim.

He was not able to participate in the decision making process. When Henry's daughter and son were asked if he had ever expressed any desires or beliefs about what he would like done for him if he were every severely incapacitated, they could not remember him saying anything about the matter.

If theoretically we think that the right balance of patient autonomy and beneficence ought to shape medical decisions, how should we think about situations like Henry's? Should the *family's* needs and preferences play a role in such cases? If you were Henry's physician, what analogies would you use to delineate the morally salient features of the case?

A third aspect of casuistry, kinetics, points out that when we have a set of very difficult cases the use of warrants, maxims and circumstances to reach a conclusion or resolution merely makes that conclusion part of the circumstances for an analogous case. There will be a useful and productive moral movement from case to case if we can incorporate well what is the prime conclusion of one case as a part of the circumstantial premises of another case and so on to a whole string of cases.

Suppose we conclude in the previous case that Henry's family has a right to make the decision about his treatment. They, after all, have to suffer the consequences of whatever decision is made. Henry really has enormously reduced autonomy and prolonging his life is not likely to benefit him in any case. We may be able to use similar reasoning to help us decide how to treat in other sorts of cases, providing the latter are similar enough to the circumstances in Henry's case.

A 23-year-old woman, Julia, was brought to the obstetrics clinic at Memorial Hospital by her mother. Julia had not had a menstrual period in 12 weeks. She was severely mentally retarded, blind and unable to communicate. Julia's mother worked ten hours a day as a waitress, and was her daughter's only means of support. Medicaid would not pay for the abortion, and there was no way to tell who had caused the pregnancy. Julia's mother was 54 years old and felt she was incapable of raising another child.

Since Julia was an adult there were no legal provisions permitting the mother to make the decision for Julia to have an abortion, unless she were made Julia's legal guardian. The mother, however, wanted Julia to have an abortion. Since Julia had been born retarded, she was worried that her baby might be as well. That would make adoption difficult if Julia came to term and delivered the baby. She did not feel she could wait for Julia to have an amniocentesis, and said she did not consider that test reliable.

It could be argued that Julia has, like every other woman, reproductive rights. But rights rest on interests, and it is not clear that Julia had a moral interest in carrying the fetus to term because of her mental status. Like Henry, she is also incapable of making a decision on her own on the basis of reasons, even bad reasons. What are the positive analogies between this case and Henry's situation? What are the negative analogies? If we consider the central feature of the previous case to be reflection on the relevant interests of all parties involved, can we use the conclusion there in at least a preliminary way to reveal the salient feature of Julia's situation?

Fourth, probability in casuistry will be higher the more we have a sort of sense of assurance in the resolution of cases. The sort of strong sense of moral satisfaction noted in the Scots tradition and in pragmatism has its special place at this stage in the casuistical tradition.

The reliance of clinical medicine and clinical medical ethics on this kind of casuistic approach is rather clearly seen in the diagnostic situation. Here a pattern of signs and symptoms is cited which contains more of the presumptive elements of one medical and ethical condition than of another. Because of this pattern we will medically and ethically prescribe measures appropriate to this condition. Should further or different signs and symptoms surface as we prognostically proceed we will be constantly alert to the possibility of a paradigm shift.[31]

This kind of ethical approach notes that the theories of biomedical science do not neatly and deductively apply to specific cases. Rather there are much more indirect and imprecise ways in which the actualities of clinical medicine are related to scientific research and theories. In clinical medicine as in clinical ethics the crucial reference points are the diseases, disabilities and injuries contained in the current taxonomy of pathological conditions. Because clinical arguments are always presumptive, not necessary, room must always be made to reach different diagnostic opinions about marginal and ambiguous cases.[32]

This casuistic approach will then stress the opportune character of timely choices and actions. There will be a strong awareness of the circumstantial dependence of ethical judgments on the detailed facts of an individual situation. Rather than searching for some abstract ethical principles the stress will be on pragmatic active involvement in pressing cases.[33] We can only find the degree of exactness or necessity the case allows. This will probably never be mathematical exactness or formal necessity. Clinical medical ethics will never be systematic in the way that abstract theoretical disciplines are. As a result clinical medical ethics cannot rest on invariable axioms or strictly universal generalizations.[34]

The practical work of clinical ethics will show a substantive rather than a formal coherence. One of the clear ways of telling whether or not a clear clinical decision has been reached is that there is a personal and team sense of conviction that the proper action is to be taken.[35] This brings in again very strongly the role of willful choice in the practice of clinical ethics. These convictions will be played out in multiple and complex contexts.

Any development of clinical ethical theories will see these as not mutually exclusive. Rather than searching for logical inconsistencies as does the professionally abstract philosopher there is an inclusive search for as many ethical approaches which can be brought to bear on the issue. Conflicting claims will better be rhetorically than logically resolved. We have to be persuaded that we are taking the best possible action.[36] As much as possible clinical ethical theories should operate as complementary practical theories each of which is relevant to some specific type of moral problem.[37]

Baruch Brody situates the working out of clinical ethical decision-making securely in the dynamics of the physician–patient relationship. He maintains that both parties are obliged to enter into a mutually understood relationship, but there are times and circumstances when overriding value considerations of the physician or patient dictate either not entering the relationship or withdrawing from it.[38] A physician who in conscience cannot be involved in abortion procedures would be such a case in point. A patient with a relatively minor complaint may decide not to seek a physician's help so as to conserve money for family purposes.

In some situations, such as the need for aggressive procedures in dealing with acute cardiac cases, the pressing medical needs of the situation may tend to override both physician and patient wishes. There are also cases of such psychological or social pressure that this may occur. Radical unavailability of funds or technology may preclude the carrying out of patient and physician wishes.[39] The physician–patient relationship must as much as possible take into account factors beyond the control of both parties and negotiate the terms of the relationship which are workable. Society has an obligation to as much as possible see to it that factors extrinsic and intrinsic to the physician–patient relationship operate smoothly. It should look to make sure that malperformance is minimized. There should also be safeguards against fraud and coercion. In certain cases society should pay for health care costs when the patient is not able to do so.[40]

This interpersonal physician–patient approach to the practical solving of clinical ethical cases is put into a casuistic type frame in that the resolution for tensions and problems is made by an appeal to a variety of ethical approaches. The more many of them can practically operate in a given case, the better the chance that our ethical convictions in the case are correct. Five ethical approaches are especially noted: a concern with the consequences of actions, an appeal to rights, a stress on respect for persons, an attempt to incorporate as many moral virtues as possible into the case, a concern for cost-effectiveness and social justice.[41]

Martha Nussbaum in her daringly creative re-working of Aristotle's approach to the virtues enumerates eight basically human factors which come into play in one way or another whenever we attempt to engage in the habitual practice of virtuous activity.[42] We have always a sense of mortality. This can and should not be a morbid dread of the inevitable but a more constructive basic awareness of the human condition. It forms an ever present horizon for all of our ethical actions. This awareness is intimately connected with another constant human experience, the sense of bodiliness. Crucial especially for medical ethics is the constant awareness of the strengths and constraints imposed on us by our biological condition.

We are biologically and psychologically always in the situation of experiencing a certain amount of pleasure and pain. Our cognitive activities and capabilities are in the context of frustration or fulfillment. We need to be able to pragmatically and practically reason our way through to workable conclusions.

Nussbaum notes that Aristotle places the practice of virtue ethics securely in the context of human interrelation and affiliation. To this she adds two other parts of the frame for ethical reasoning. One is the rooting of human affiliation in early infantile experience. Here she admits readily the influence of Freud. The other is an unusual noting of the necessary place of humor in ethical reasoning. This may at first seem very strange indeed, but the peculiar human ability to note incongruities which is the very heart of humor also is a sign of the imperfect and incomplete context in which we ethically muddle toward some kind of resolution. Even ethicists should learn not to take themselves too terribly seriously.

The hypothetical character of moral reasoning is stressed

by Philippa Foot, another pioneer in the current renewal of the theory and practice of virtue ethics.[43] The book is dedicated to Iris Murdoch, the prolific novelist and philosopher. In a classic work Murdoch describes the narrative patterns of a person's progressing life as the setting for an ethics of virtue.[44] Bernard Williams notes that these patterns of living regularly involve instances of sheer luck. He thinks that there is such a thing as moral luck so that we sometimes have a better, sometimes a worse chance of reaching a really satisfactory ethical decision.[45] What gives a certain permanence and continuity to ethics is a set of personally felt dispositions or drives which move us toward the degree of ethical resolution possible in any given situation. But he is quite stringent on the limits to the possibilities of problematic solutions.[46] James D. Wallace, taking his cue from John Dewey, strongly points out the importance of the network of personal interests and relationships in which the habitual patterns of virtue ethics can flourish.[47]

The work of Edmund Pellegrino and David Thomasma may provide the final framework in which we wish to explore the workings of virtue ethics. This because they explicitly map out the context for virtuous activity in the practice of clinical medical ethics. Pellegrino notes three basic moments in medical ethical decision-making. The first, the diagnostic, tries to respond to what can be wrong. It is an attempt to isolate the source of the medical and ethical problem. The second, the therapeutic, is a response to the question as to what can be done. The third component, the prudential, involves the search for a right answer to the problem of a specific patient.[48]

In further work with Thomasma the concern for the individual patient, called beneficence-in-trust, focuses on four aspects of the patient's good.[49] The first is a general view of the ultimate meaning of life and human destiny as perceived by the patient. This could be either a religious or more secular sense of the situation of one's self in the order of things. It would be very important in life and death decisions to be as much in harmony with this as possible. Second, we must respect and cater to the freedom of the patient or patient's family. We should foster as much possibility for free choice on their part as is possible in the constrained circumstances of disease or illness.

Third, we should listen to patient preferences in terms of their own perceived quality of life. We should not be too aggressive in attempting to change or influence the patients' own life plans, goals

171

and aims into which medical intervention fits as only one part or aspect. Finally, the biomedical or clinical diagnostic and therapeutic indications must be fitted prudentially in the frame of the patients' larger scheme of perceived priorities and values.

On the patients' side there ought to be a concern to tell the truth, to be compliant about agreed upon steps to recovery or palliation, also an avoidance of manipulation of physicians and other health professionals.[50]

The mutual cooperation and trust that would then be set up in physician-patient relationships would provide the nurturing framework in which we might experience and practice the creative complexities of virtue ethics to the best possible benefit of our medical and ethical health.

NOTES

INTRODUCTION: ETHICAL PRACTICE IN CLINICAL MEDICINE

1 W. D. Ross, *The Right and the Good* (Oxford: Oxford University Press, 1930), 21.
2 R. C. Sider and C. D. Clements, "The New Medical Ethics: a Second Opinion," *Archives of Internal Medicine*, 145 (December, 1985), 2169–71; and C. D. Clements and R. C. Sider, "Medical Ethics' Assault on Medical Values," *Journal of the American Medical Association*, 250 (October, 1983), 2011–15.
3 G. Engel, "The Need for a New Medical Model: A Challenge for Biomedicine," *Science* 196 (1977), 129–36; and G. Engel, "The Clinical Application of the Biopsychosocial Model," *American Journal of Psychiatry*, 137 (May, 1980), 535–44.

1 THE PLATONIC FOUNDATION

1 The texts of Plato will be cited using the standard marginal notations. In this case: 68a–69d.
2 190c–194c
3 195d
4 198a
5 330a
6 349d
7 361abc
8 70a–71b
9 73b
10 79e
11 89a
12 89a
13 96b
14 100a
15 253de
16 503c

17 258bc
18 296bc
19 306bc
20 653b
21 661a–662e
22 696a–697c
23 733e
24 905e–906a
25 906c
26 967d

2 THE ARISTOTELIAN FRAME

1 The texts of Aristotle will be cited using the standard marginal notations, in this case 1259 b 20
2 1260 a 10
3 1260 a 5
4 1325 b 15
5 1334 a 20
6 1102 b 10
7 1102 a 30
8 1103 a 5
9 1130 b 30
10 1101 b 30
11 1103 a 25
12 1103 a 30
13 1104 a 10
14 1104 a 25
15 1109 a 25
16 1105 b 1
17 1105 b 15
18 1106 a 10
19 1139 a 30
20 1140 a 30
21 1140 b 5
22 1140 a 25
23 1155 b 20
24 1156 a 5–1156 b 5
25 1156 b 5–1156 b 30

3 THOMISTIC PRUDENCE

1 The so-called "treatise on the virtues" in the *Summa Theologiae* is in the first part of the second section of this large work. Since all of the book is written in the question and answer style peculiar to medieval scholasticism, the material is handled in several questions which are subdivided into articles. The standard abbreviated way of referring to

these questions and articles will be used. For instance, the present citation is q.49, a.1.

2 q.49, a.2.
3 q.49, a.3.
4 q.49, a.4.
5 q.51, a.1.
6 q.51, a.2.
7 q.51, a.3.
8 q.53, a.1.
9 q.54, a.4.
10 q.55, a.1.
11 q.55, a.2.
12 q.55, a.4.
13 q.56, a.1.
14 q.56, a.3.
15 q.56, a.4.
16 q.56, a.6.
17 q.57, a.1.
18 q.57, a.2.
19 q.57, a.4.
20 q.58, a.3.
21 q.58, a.4.
22 q.58, a.5.
23 q.61, a.2.

4 SCOTTISH MORAL SENSE

1 On this matter with particular relation to the work of Jefferson see: Garry Wills, *Inventing America*, (Garden City, New York: Doubleday and Company, Inc.). I am deeply indebted to the work of my colleague Professor Mark Waymack for a good deal of the perspectives on some of the Scottish philosophers here treated. Mark H. Waymack, "Moral Philosophy and Newtonianism in the Scottish Enlightenment: A Study of the Moral Philosophies of Gershom Carmichael, Francis Hutcheson, David Hume and Adam Smith," diss., Johns Hopkins University, 1986.
2 Francis Hutcheson, *Collected Works*, 7 vols (Hildesheim, 1969–71) 1 *An Inquiry into the Original of our Ideas of Beauty and Virtue*, (1725) 173, and 2 *An Essay on the Nature and Conduct of the Passions and Affectations, with Illustrations upon the Moral Sense*, 2 (1728) 216.
3 Hutcheson, *Inquiry*, 15.
4 ibid., 92–3.
5 Hutcheson, *Illustrations*, 216.
6 ibid., 217.
7 Joseph Butler, *Works of Joseph Butler*, vol. 2 *The Sermons* (Oxford: Clarendon Press, 1896) 187–8.
8 The strong regulatory and epistemic quality of emotive factors is well brought out in a recent article by Sidney Callahan, "The Role of

Emotion in Decisionmaking," *Hastings Center Report* 18.3 (1988) 9–14.
9 Hutcheson, *Inquiry*, 128.
10 Francis Hutcheson, *Collected Works* 7 vols (Hildesheim, 1969–71) vols 5–6, *System of Moral Philosophy* 1.
11 Hutcheson, *System of Moral Philosophy* 19–20, 25–8.
12 Francis Hutcheson, *Collected Works*, 7 vols (Hildesheim, 1969–71), vol. 4 *A Short Introduction to Moral Philosophy* 61–2.
13 David Hume, *A Treatise of Human Nature*, ed. Nidditch (Oxford: Clarendon Press, 1978) 577.
14 Hume, *Treatise of Human Nature*, 580.
15 ibid., 479.
16 ibid., 575.
17 ibid., 587.
18 Adam Smith, *The Wealth of Nations* (Chicago: University of Chicago Press, 1976) The invisible hand quote appears in Book IV, chapter 2.
19 Adam Smith, *The Theory of Moral Sentiments*, ed. A. L. Macfie and D. D. Raphael (Oxford: Clarendon Press, 1976), I.i.4.2.
20 Adam Smith, *Essays on Philosophical Subjects*, ed. W. P. D. Wightman (Oxford: Clarendon Press, 1976) 42.
21 Smith, *Theory of Moral Sentiments*, I.i.3.9.
22 ibid., VII.iii.3.16.
23 ibid., VI.i.5.
24 ibid., II.ii.3.2–3.
25 ibid., VI.iii.3.1.
26 Thomas Reid, *Essays on the Active Powers of the Human Mind*, (Cambridge: MIT Press, 1969) 462.
27 Reid, *Active Powers*, 35.
28 ibid., 361–7.
29 ibid., 85.
30 ibid., 86.
31 ibid., 88.
32 ibid., 151–3.
33 ibid., 210.
34 ibid., 208.
35 ibid., 204.
36 ibid., 215.
37 ibid., 224–5.
38 ibid., 390.

5 AMERICAN PRAGMATISM

1 Diary entry quoted in Ralph Barton Perry, *The Thought and Character of William James*, 2 vols (Boston: Little, Brown, 1935) vol. 1, 323.
2 William James, "The Moral Philosopher and the Moral Life," in *The Will to Believe, and Other Essays in Popular Philosophy* (New York: Dover, 1956) 213–15.
3 William James, *The Principles of Psychology*, 2 vols (New York: Dover, 1950) 672.

4 William James "On a Certain Blindness in Human Beings," in *Talks to Teachers* (New York: Norton, 1958) 149.
5 James, *Talks to Teachers*, 165.
6 James, *Principles of Psychology*, 288.
7 William James, *The Letters of William James*, ed. Henry James III, 2 vols (New York: Kraus Reprint Co., 1969) 1: 127–33.
8 William James, "German Pessimism," in *Collected Essays and Reviews* (New York: Russell and Russell, 1969) 18.
9 William James, *Pragmatism* (Cambridge: Harvard University Press, 1975) 185.
10 James, "The Moral Philosopher and the Moral Life," 187.
11 ibid., 195.
12 James, *Principles of Psychology*, 2:315.
13 James, "The Moral Philosopher and the Moral Life," 213.
14 Jo Ann Boydston, ed., *The Study of Ethics: A Syllabus*, by John Dewey, vol. 4 of *John Dewey: The Early Works, 1893–1894* (Carbondale: Southern Illinois University Press, 1971) 223.
15 Dewey, *Study of Ethics*, 235.
16 Jo Ann Boydston, ed., "The Reflex Arc Concept in Psychology," in vol. 5 of *John Dewey: The Early Works, 1882–1889* (Carbondale: Southern Illinois University Press) 97.
17 Jo Ann Boydston, ed., *Ethics*, by John Dewey and Jame Tufts, vol. 5 of *John Dewey: The Middle Works, 1899–1924* (Carbondale: Southern Illinois University Press, 1978); and Jo Ann Boydston, ed., *Ethics*, by John Dewey and James Tufts, vol. 7 of *John Dewey: The Later Works, 1925–1953* (Carbondale: Southern Illinois University Press 1985).
18 Dewey and Tufts, 1908 *Ethics*, 326.
19 ibid., 359.
20 Dewey and Tufts, 1932 *Ethics*, 327.
21 John Dewey, "Trois facteurs indépendants en matière de morale," trans. Charles Cestre, in *Bulletin de la société française de philosophie* 30 (October–December 1930): 118–27, from an address read in English before the French Philosophical Society, Paris, November 7, 1930. First published in English in *Educational Theory* 16 (July 1966): trans. Jo Ann Boydston. Also in Jo Ann Boydston, ed., *Individualism, Old and New*, by John Dewey, vol. 5 of *John Dewey: The Later Works, 1925–1953* (Carbondale: Southern Illinois University Press, 1981) 279–88.
22 Dewey and Tufts, 1932 *Ethics*, xxxii.
23 ibid., xxxiv.
24 ibid., 182.
25 ibid., 163–4.
26 ibid., 168.
27 ibid., 164.
28 ibid., 166.
29 ibid., 167.
30 ibid., 170–1.
31 ibid., 243–5.
32 ibid., 247–8.
33 ibid., 256–7.

34 ibid., 258–9.
35 ibid., 187.
36 ibid., 210.
37 ibid., 218.
38 ibid., 276.
39 ibid., 277.
40 ibid., 277–8.
41 ibid., 280–1.
42 ibid., 179–80.

6 CONTEMPORARY DEVELOPMENTS IN VIRTUE ETHICS

1 Collen D. Clements and Roger S. Sider, "Medical Ethics' Assault Upon Medical Values," *Journal of the American Medical Association* 250 (1983): 2015.
2 Collen D. Clements and Roger C. Sider, "The New Medical Ethics: a Second Opinion," *Archives of Internal Medicine* 145 (1985): 2169.
3 Edward O. Wilson, *The Insect Societies* (Cambridge, Massachusetts: Belknap Press of Harvard University Press, 1971) 322.
4 Wilson, *The Insect Societies* 460.
5 Edward O. Wilson, *Sociobiology: the New Synthesis* (Cambridge, Massachusetts: Belknap Press of Harvard University Press, 1975) 4.
6 Wilson, *Sociobiology*, 552.
7 Edward O. Wilson, *On Human Nature* (New York: Bantam Books, 1982) 70.
8 Wilson, *On Human Nature*, 162.
9 Charles J. Lumsden and Edward O. Wilson, *Genes, Mind and Culture* (Cambridge, Massachusetts: Harvard University Press, 1981) 370.
10 Lumsden and Wilson, *Genes, Mind, and Culture*, 368.
11 Edward O. Wilson, *Biophilia* (Cambridge, Massachusetts: Harvard University Press, 1984) 138–9.
12 Wilson, *Biophilia*, 67, 74, 100–1.
13 Gunther S. Stent, "The Poverty of Scientism and the Promise of Structuralist Ethics," *The Hastings Center Report* 6.6 (1976): 32–40.
14 Gunther S. Stent, *Paradoxes of Progress* (San Francisco: W. H. Freeman and Company, 1978).
15 Leon R. Kass, M.D., *Toward a More Natural Science: Biology and Human Affairs* (New York: The Free Press, 1985) 265.
16 Kass, *Toward a More Natural Science*, 274–5.
17 ibid. 311–14.
18 Ernst Mayr, *Evolution and the Diversity of Life* (Cambridge, Massachusetts: The Belknap Press of Harvard University Press, 1976) 403.
19 The material in this section is taken from Erik H. Erikson, *Identity and the Life Cycle* (New York: Norton, 1980).
20 Kohlberg tended to publish or circulate his material in articles rather than fully finished books. Two such articles which might be of considerable help are: Lawrence Kohlberg, "Stages of Development as

a Basis for Moral Education," in *Moral Education: Interdisciplinary Approaches*, ed. C. M. Beck, B. S. Crittenden, and E. V. Sullivan (Toronto: University of Toronto Press, 1971) and Lawrence Kohlberg, "Moral Stages and Moralization: The Cognitive-Developmental Approach," in *Moral Development and Behavior*, ed. Thomas Lickona (New York: Holt, Rinehart and Winston, 1976).

21 John Rawls, *A Theory of Justice* (Cambridge, Massachusetts: The Belknap Press of Harvard University Press, 1971) 30.

22 Rawls, *A Theory of Justice*, 195–200.

23 Norman Daniels, *Just Health Care* (Cambridge: Cambridge University Press, 1988) 42–8.

24 John Finnis, *Natural Law and Natural Rights* (Oxford: Clarendon Press, 1980) 100–27.

25 Alasdair MacIntyre, *After Virtue* (Notre Dame, Indiana: University of Notre Dame Press, 1981) 169–89.

26 Adapted from the remarks of Ruth Purtilo at the Second National Conference on Ethics Consultation in Health Care, St. Louis, Missouri, September 22–4, 1988.

27 Albert A. Jonsen, "On Being a Casuist," in *Clinical Medical Ethics: Exploration and Assessment* (Lanham, Maryland: University Press of America, 1987) 119–24.

28 Albert R. Jonsen and Stephen Toulmin, *The Abuse of Casuistry* (Berkeley and Los Angeles, California: University of California Press, 1988) 27.

29 Jonsen and Toulmin, *The Abuse of Casuistry*, 34–5.

30 Albert Jonsen, "The Place of Ethics in Ethics Consultation," The Second National Conference on Ethics Consultation in Health Care, St. Louis, Missouri, September 23, 1988.

31 Jonsen and Toulmin, *The Abuse of Casuistry*, 41.

32 ibid., 43.

33 ibid., 67.

34 ibid., 281.

35 ibid., 286.

36 ibid., 295.

37 ibid., 298.

38 Baruch Brody, *Life and Death Decision Making* (New York: Oxford University Press, 1988) 73.

39 Brody, *Life and Death Decision Making*, 73.

40 ibid.

41 ibid., 79–94.

42 Martha Nussbaum, "Non–Relative Virtues: An Aristotelian Approach," in Peter A. French, Theodore E. Uehling, Jr., and Howard K. Wettstein, eds, *Midwest Studies in Philosophy v. XIII, Ethical Theory: Character and Virtue* (Notre Dame, Indiana: University of Notre Dame Press, 1988) 48–9.

43 Philippa Foot, *Virtues and Vices And Other Essays in Moral Philosophy* (Berkeley: University of California Press, 1978) 164–7.

44 Iris Murdoch, *The Sovereignty of Good* (London: Routledge and Kegan Paul, 1970) 26.

45 Bernard Williams, *Moral Luck* (Cambridge: Cambridge University Press, 1981) 20–39.
46 Bernard Williams, *Ethics and the Limits of Philosophy* (Cambridge, Massachusetts: Harvard University Press, 1985) 50–1.
47 James D. Wallace, *Moral Relevance and Moral Conflict* (Ithaca, New York: Cornell University Press, 1988) 76.
48 Edmund Pellegrino, "The Anatomy of Clinical Judgments: Some Notes on Right Reason and Right Action," in H. T. Engelhardt, Jr. *et al.*, eds, *Clinical Judgment: A Critical Appraisal* (Boston and Dordrecht: D. Reidel Publishing Company, 1979) 174.
49 Edmund C. Pellegrino and David C. Thomasma, *For the Patient's Good: the Restoration of Beneficence in Health Care* (New York: Oxford University Press, 1988) 81–2.
50 Pellegrino and Thomasma, *For the Patient's Good*, 106.

INDEX

hemophilia 120
heroism 95
hierarchy of medicine 21–3, 35, 134–5
higher life forms 139
history 126
HIV status 68–9, 98, 120, 122–3
Hobbes, Thomas 154
holiness 8
honesty 90
honor 90
hope 101, 102, 103
hours of working 36
household management 20–1
human affiliation 170
human experience 25, 28
human experimentation 17–18, 70
human nature 30, 41
Human Nature and Conduct (Dewey) 107
Hume, David 75–6
humility 75
humor 170
Huntington's chorea 9–10
Hutcheson, Francis 64–74 *passim*, 85

ideal of goodness 14, 15
idealism 6, 13, 15, 45, 83
ideals, ethical 12–13, 69–70
identity crisis 142
imagination 80, 86, 136–7
immortality 139
imperfection 96–7
impulse 105–7, 113, 122, 125, 137
individuals 23, 72, 76, 130–1
industry–inferiority crisis 142
infantile experience 170
inferiority 142
informed consent 18, 24, 124, 164
initiative 142
inner drives 38, 50–1, 53–5, 73, 90, 113
insect societies 130, 131
instinct, reason and 38
instinctive emotions 88–9, 90
Institute for the Medical Humanities 147, 156
integrity 142

intellect, will and 49, 50, 51
intellectual: habits 57; knowledge 26, 30, 40, 60; principles 50; reasoning 86–7; virtues 28–30
intelligence 108
intended act 165
intentionality 58–61, 165
internal goods 158
interpersonal interactions 81–3
interpersonal relationships 149, 154–5; physician–patient 2, 9, 59, 70, 72–5, 81–3, 169–72
intimacy 142
"invisible hand" 76, 78
irascible appetite 51, 52
irrational drives 142
isolation 142

James, W. 4, 10, 91–105, 128
Jehovah's Witnesses 24, 83–4
Jonsen, A.R. 162–3
Journal of the American Medical Association 4, 128
juridical decisions 126
justice: Aquinas on 54, 61; Aristotelian 23, 25–6, 27; contemporary development 132, 147, 154; moral sense 71–3, 75–6, 84–5, 90; Platonic 8, 12, 15; *prima facie* 3, 4, 154
justifying reasons 73

Kant, Immanuel 153
Kass, Leon 5, 139
kinetics 167
kinship 130
knowledge 6, 7, 8, 16; abstract 89; and beliefs 85; in decision-making 115–16; ethical 63; growth 40–1; habitual 29; intellectual 26, 30, 40, 60; medical 57–61; practical 10, 12–13, 32–7, 40–4, 163; of principles 57–8, 61; quest for 70; sense 26, 63; skilled 89
Kohlberg, L. 5, 146–9, 152

L-Dopa 10
Laches (Plato) 7